YOUR
BIRTH PLAN

YOUR
BIRTH PLAN

A GUIDE TO NAVIGATING ALL OF YOUR CHOICES IN CHILDBIRTH

Megan Davidson

ROWMAN & LITTLEFIELD
Lanham • Boulder • New York • London

Published by Rowman & Littlefield
An imprint of The Rowman & Littlefield Publishing Group, Inc.
4501 Forbes Boulevard, Suite 200, Lanham, Maryland 20706
www.rowman.com

6 Tinworth Street, London, SE11 5AL, United Kingdom

Distributed by NATIONAL BOOK NETWORK

All photos are courtesy of the author.

This book contains information about health care but it represents reference material only. This book is not a medical manual and should not be used in lieu of consulting with trained medical professionals. The data presented here are meant to assist the reader in making informed choices in consultation with their clinical care team, never as a replacement for appropriate prenatal care with doctor or midwife. Mention of particular medications, products, or authorities in this book does not entail endorsement by the publisher or author. Both the author and publisher disclaim any liability for medical outcomes related to applying the information suggested here to your health care.

British Library Cataloguing in Publication Information Available

Library of Congress Cataloging-in-Publication Data

Names: Davidson, Megan, 1977– author.
Title: Your birth plan : a guide to navigating all of your choices in childbirth / Megan Davidson.
Description: Lanham : Rowman & Littlefield, [2019] | Includes bibliographical references and index.
Identifiers: LCCN 2018049542 (print) | LCCN 2018052967 (ebook) | ISBN 9781538121580 (electronic) | ISBN 9781538121573 (pbk. : alk. paper)
Subjects: LCSH: Pregnancy—Popular works. | Childbirth—Popular works.
Classification: LCC RG525 (ebook) | LCC RG525 .D318 2019 (print) | DDC 618.2—dc23
LC record available at https://lccn.loc.gov/2018049542

∞™ The paper used in this publication meets the minimum requirements of American National Standard for Information Sciences—Permanence of Paper for Printed Library Materials, ANSI/NISO Z39.48-1992.

Printed in the United States of America

With enormous thanks to all the families
who have shared their births with me,

and for August and Clay,
who taught me about the power of a positive birth.

CONTENTS

PREFACE
My Birth Story

At the University of New Mexico in the late 1990s, I had the great fortune to study with Rina Swentzell, a Santa Clara Pueblo architect, historian, potter, and visiting professor at UNM. She taught for only one semester while I was there but was one of my most influential teachers. Rina reminded me of my mother: she was beautiful, soft spoken, and kind. At the end of the semester she gifted us each a handmade piece of pottery. My present was a pueblo mudhead that sits on a shelf in my kitchen still.

In her seminar, Rina prompted us to explore oral traditions and storytelling. Instead of writing a final paper drawn from published texts and known experts, Rina challenged us to find a storyteller and tell their story. I knew immediately the story I wanted to tell.

My mother has written in diaries and journals her entire life. For my final project, I relied on the notes she wrote before and after my birth—complete with doodled name options in the margins, a grocery list (batteries, strawberries, envelopes), and child care plans for my brothers contingent on when labor began. She'd written about finding out she was pregnant, her hopes and fears as she approached motherhood again, her struggle with the hospital to ensure they would respect her wishes for the birth, and later, the triumph of giving birth. Drawing from her notes, I wrote my birth story.

Five days before I was born, on the estimated due date given by her doctor, she wrote about cramping and vomiting during the night. She'd hoped this was labor beginning, but it wasn't. A jeweler, she wrote about a ruby and sapphire sale at her store and an opal ring she'd sold. She wrote about an employee she might hire. She said her doctor was on call that weekend and going into labor that night would be perfect. She wrote the word "pickles" in the margin.

The next entry is from the day after I was born. It begins with her writing that she's at home with Megan asleep on her legs, an experience she described as "far out" (I was born in the late 1970s). While I'm the fourth child in my family, I'm the only girl and my mom didn't know this before I was born. She wrote that during the brief moment of birth—the short space between when my head was born and the rest of my body came out—she'd wanted to wait, holding on to the possibility of having a girl a few seconds more. My umbilical cord briefly fooled her, but she wrote she was now confident she was finally the mother of a daughter.

Her labor with me was "pretty easy," even though I was the biggest of her babies and the labor was both longer and stronger than her last birth. Less than six hours after her water broke in the farmhouse my parents owned at the time, she gave birth. The hospital respected the list of demands she sent them months earlier, insisting she didn't want a repeat of any of the less favorable parts of her last birth. She birthed me outside of an operating room (no longer common but operating room births were the norm), with my dad present, using Lamaze breathing techniques. She was discharged the same day and felt great because she'd had a strong voice in the process.

Five years after I took Rina's class, living in New York and finishing my master's degree in anthropology, I was eight months pregnant and preparing for my own birth. I'd found supportive care providers whom I trusted. My husband, Shawn, and I had taken a childbirth education class. I'd reread my mother's stories about her births for inspiration and insights.

After months of planning and preparing for our future child, in mid-July, a few days after the estimated due date they'd given me, contractions began. I remember I'd asked everyone what contractions would feel like and how I'd know when labor started. The replies were vague with lots of reassurance that I'd know. I was frustrated by these responses, but when I had the first real contractions of my labor, I did immediately know. After weeks of funny feelings and wondering, *Is this it?*, by the second contraction I was certain I was in labor. I remember smiling to myself as I paced the long hallway in our apartment, realizing everyone had been right.

Giving birth to our son, August, was at once one of the absolute best experiences of my life and also the hardest thing I'd ever done. I felt like nothing I'd done to date compared to the experience in terms of both physical and emotional intensity. Prior to giving birth, I'd worked as a rape crisis and domestic violence advocate, first in New Mexico and then in New York, including working on another floor of the hospital I was now laboring in. I wished for the type

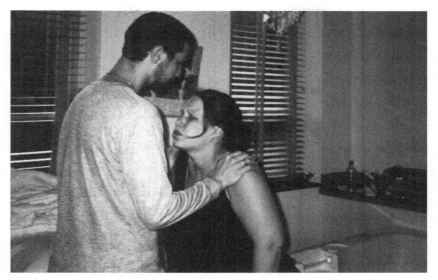

In labor with my first child, August.

of support I offered survivors and their families as Shawn and I navigated a long labor and all the anxiety and challenges that came with it.

My birth taught me so much about the value of support, reassurance, guidance, and help in childbirth, and it led me to become a doula. A doula is a professional birth support person who provides physical, emotional, and informational support throughout pregnancy, labor, birth, and the postpartum period. I'm a non–medical professional, but I understand the medical aspects of birth and I use this knowledge to help my clients understand what's happening and what their options are. I work to reduce fear and build confidence, increase knowledge and informed decision-making, advocate for my clients during labor and birth, offer physical support for coping with labor, and help to ensure that the experience of their birth is a positive one. I also work with people extensively in the first months after giving birth, offering guidance with feeding, healing, newborn care, and the emotional impact of parenthood. I don't advocate for any specific type of birth or experiences. Instead, I advocate for people to be treated with respect, to be informed, to be able to make their *own* decisions, and to have positive experiences of childbirth.

One year after August was born, I finished the coursework and exams for my PhD and no longer needed to live near Binghamton University while I researched and wrote my dissertation. We moved to Fort Greene, Brooklyn. In

2007, I finished my PhD and I gave birth to our second son, Clay. My graduation was on a Sunday, the day before my due date, but driving hours upstate for the ceremony seemed both unwise and uncomfortable. Instead, we threw a huge party.

My sister-in-law, Melissa, was the last person to arrive at the party. She took a cab straight from the airport to be there. She and Aaron, my oldest brother, live five blocks away and we're very close. I'd invited Melissa to be with us for the birth because she'd never been to a birth and we agreed it would be a special experience. I was aware the week before my due date that she was abroad for work, and I didn't want to give birth until she returned. Before she left the party that night, Melissa bent down and spoke to my belly, saying: "I am back! You can come out anytime now. Thanks for waiting for me." I laughed and joked that I would call her at 4:00 a.m.

Shawn and I fell asleep around midnight. I woke up at 3:30 a.m., as usual, needing to pee. As I left the bathroom, I felt a familiar sensation—a contraction, a real one. I lay back down hoping for more sleep, but another contraction came, affirming what I suspected: labor had begun. I woke Shawn to let him know and labored quietly to let August sleep. My mom was in town to help with August, and she took him to my brother's house after breakfast. They alerted Melissa that today was the day, and she came over with a box of groceries and prepared one of my favorite meals. About fifteen hours after that first contraction, our son Clay was born in another positive birth experience where I felt safe, supported, cared for, and respected.

One afternoon later that year, on a local city bus with my sons, I noted with great pleasure that one of the quotes memorialized on the side of a Brooklyn building was from Rina Swentzell. We got off the bus immediately. I stood on the sidewalk reading her words to my children:

> What we are told as children is people when they walk on the land leave their breath wherever they go. So wherever we walk, that particular spot on the earth never forgets us, and when we go back to these places, we know that the people who have lived there are in some way still there, and that we can actually partake of their breath and their spirit.

I've passed this quote often on my way to prenatal visits and postpartum appointments with expectant and new parents. I've passed this quote in the middle of the night as I travel to join laboring clients in their homes. I've sat stuck at a red light in a cab on the way to the hospital with a person in labor on hands and knees moaning through contractions with Rina's quote illuminated on the

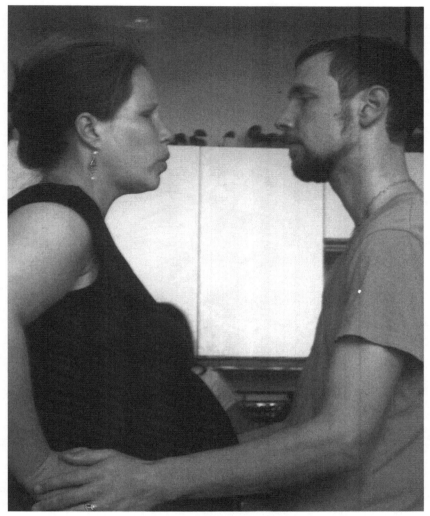

In labor with my second child, Clay.

side of the road next to us. I remind my client to exhale, and let her breath help her relax through the contraction or enjoy the space in between. I think about her breath and how she is leaving it here as part of the story of giving birth. I think about Rina and my mother and the path that brought me to motherhood, being a doula, and writing this book.

For me, this book is an intervention into how we think about and prepare for childbirth. You will not find a childbirth method here. There is no prescription for what you should think or want or eat or practice while you're pregnant. There are no recipes, meditations, herbal tinctures, or descriptions of how you should feel. I'm not offering a branded technique to practice in pregnancy for comfort during labor. You are yourself—the same person you've always been—and you likely don't need to radically reorder who you are in order to have this baby.

That said, you likely do need information to make choices about where you are going to give birth, who you are going to have with you on your birth team, and what it looks like for you to have a positive experience of giving birth. That is what you'll find here. I present grounded, thoughtful, evidence-based information about all options without judgment or prescription to help you make the best decisions for yourself. I draw from my experience of helping nearly six hundred people give birth in hospitals, birth centers, and every type of NYC home with the care of hundreds of different doctors and midwives and with every type of preference, intervention, and outcome available. My clients and many other new parents generously shared their stories, experiences, and thoughts to help in the creation of this book.

I also extensively researched up-to-date medical data to provide the most accurate information available. That said, it's worth noting that medicine is a field where things change: new studies come out, new medicines are created or older medicines are used in novel ways, different techniques gain popularity, or litigation creates practice changes, for better or worse. I've taken care to be truthful and to represent the best of our knowledge, both clinically and in the experiences I've shared, both my clients' and my own.

I want to help you have a good experience of childbirth, free from judgment and without apologizing for what you want and need from this experience. Most people remember giving birth for the rest of their lives, and whatever that looks like for you, I want you to be able to remember it as a positive experience.

INTRODUCTION

Birth Like That

"**I**'m sorry."

Jo looked at me from her hospital bed—fetal heart-rate monitors strapped to her belly, an IV pumping fluid into her vein, an epidural catheter delivering pain medication into her lower back. "I'm sorry," she said. Confused, I asked her what she was sorry for. She'd just gotten an epidural—something she'd originally wanted to avoid—and was resting for the first time in hours. She looked peaceful.

"Do you regret getting the epidural?" I asked her.

"No, not at all," Jo said. "I feel great."

"You made a good decision, one that was right for you," I told her. "Do not apologize to me—don't apologize to anyone! Don't apologize for having a birth you feel good about."

Jo's words were not new to me. During their births, I hear clients apologize for their choices, for their bodies, for being emotional, for being in pain, for making sounds, for their birth being a slow or messy process, for not understanding medical terminology or being confused, for needing help, for having questions. All things they don't need to apologize for. I understand that apologizing is often a way of being polite and it might be a deeply ingrained response, as it often is for me. I want to suggest, though, that it's OK to *not* apologize in your birth. It's OK to want what you want, whatever that is, and not owe anyone an explanation or apology.

You can have a homebirth in your living room even though other people might tell you that you're reckless. You can schedule a Cesarean birth even though others might tell you Cesareans are to be avoided whenever possible.

You might want to get an epidural and watch TV in labor even though others might tell you that unmedicated birth was transformative for them. You might opt for no pain medications even though people might tell you to stop being a martyr and there are no medals. This is your birth, your way.

That said, you might find that very little in your life up until this point has prepared you for the decisions and plans you need to make for birth. You might not know what you want or how to get it. Birth is so minimally taught or talked about in most of our lives that it's not uncommon to find yourself pregnant with little knowledge about what comes next or the consequences of the decisions you need to make in early pregnancy.

Many of us are steeped in the fictions presented on TV or in movies about what birth might look like, and we have to unlearn much of that. Add to that the enormous amounts of opinions from friends, family, neighbors, strangers, and experts about the "right way" or the "best way" to give birth. This process can be both empowering and overwhelming. The information available can be helpful and informative or biased, judgmental, unclear, and shifting.

Part of what's confusing is that there is not just one way to birth a baby and feel good about the experience. Because no one-size-fits-all set of choices leads each person to a positive birth experience—the path to a positive birth is not prescribed or dictated—this book presents all your options so that you can make your *own* decisions.

I talked to hundreds of pregnant people and new parents while writing this book, many of whom responded to posts on social media asking to speak with people who had a positive birth experience. My posts specified I was looking for the widest range of birth experiences including "birth centers, hospitals, homebirths, OBs, midwives, doulas, first baby or not, pain medication or none, induction or spontaneous, twins or singletons, vaginal or Cesarean birth." Yet, the initial responses, while valuable and appreciated, largely came from people who had a homebirth with a midwife. Two stories were even homebirths of breech babies. Homebirths are not common in the US, and vaginal breech births are even more rare; the combination is almost unheard of and I'd already collected *two* of these stories. Something was wrong.

When Theresa agreed to be interviewed, she admitted she'd seen my previous calls but assumed it was not for stories like hers, even as she described her birth as one of the best experiences of her life. In pregnancy she'd read birth stories, and while these stories were tremendously important in helping her understand what might happen and what was possible, they were also intimidating. Laughing, she told me they left her feeling like if she wasn't having an orgasm or feeling mystical during labor, she was doing it wrong. She imagined I only wanted stories from people who had birthed like that.

A GOOD BIRTH, A POSITIVE BIRTH

Theresa gave birth to her son in a hospital, with an obstetrician (OB) and an epidural (like the vast majority of people in the US), and she didn't imagine I was interested in her story. This sense of which birth stories I'd be interested in is owed in part to the concept of "natural" childbirth. I'm not sure there's consensus on what this term means: Any vaginal birth? Any birth without pain medication? Any birth without intervention? What counts or disqualifies you from this category? I suspect different people use the term in different ways, but I opt out of the term altogether because I think it suggests a hierarchy of birthing options and needs. If a natural childbirth is a vaginal birth without pain medication or intervention, are all the other ways we give birth unnatural?

This is a false, unhelpful, and disempowering framing of birth; in this book I totally reject it. Giving birth vaginally without pain medication can be an absolutely incredible experience; giving birth vaginally with pain medication, or having a surgical birth, can also be an absolutely incredible experience and should not be seen as "less than."

Birth is universally marked as a significant event: at once a biological, social, emotional, and often medical or surgical event. No matter how we get there, birth is the origin story of who we are—as parents, as people. As such, how we talk about and feel about our births matters.

When people interview me to be their doula, they often have hopes, fears, plans, and questions about their upcoming birth. I remind them that I can't promise a certain type of birth; no one can make this promise. No one can entirely alter the unpredictability of birth and ensure that an intervention isn't needed or that a baby arrives according to plan. What I can and do promise, however, is that I'll help in any way I can to make sure they feel safe, supported, respected, and heard; that I'll be with them and help them not feel afraid or alone; that I'll work to ensure they understand their options and are able to make choices and give true informed consent; and that I'll advocate for and honor their decisions, coping strategies, and needs without judgment throughout pregnancy, birth, and postpartum period. For me, this is the promise of making every effort possible to help someone have a *positive birth*. That's my goal.

A positive birth is not about having a particular type of experience or outcome per se. It can be hugely different for each person because what matters to each of us in our lives and in our births is different. My clients range enormously in what they want prenatally and how they experience their births. When I talk to pregnant clients about their "best-case scenario," or when I query new parents about what a positive birth means to them after they've given birth, the range of feelings, goals, and outcomes varies enormously.

I use the phrase "positive birth" as a way of divorcing what it means to have a good birth from the specifics of how, where, and with whom we choose to give birth. New parents and birth workers have probably all heard the phrase "healthy mother, healthy baby" spoken in reference to what the priorities of everyone's birthing should be. These words are unfortunately often used in a way that dismisses the hopes, plans, or feelings of the new parents. We all agree that having a healthy experience is an absolute priority, but you can also want to have your hopes and fears and desires respected and cared for in the process. A positive birth minds the whole picture of birth not simply as a biologic act, but also as a social and emotional experience.

THE THREE CS: CONTROL, CHOICE, CONSENT

A few years after I became a doula, I became certified as a childbirth educator. Part of that training involved mapping out classes we imagined teaching. Most of my classmates structured classes filled with statistics, problems with interventions, and fears about Cesarean birth. They crafted mantras and breathing exercises and visualizations for their imagined future students.

After years of working as a doula, I'd heard a lot of feedback from clients about what they benefited from most in their childbirth classes and also what they found silly, judgmental, or unhelpful. When I imagined the information I wanted to share, I wrote out my three Cs of childbirth: control, choice, and consent. You'll have a lot of opportunities to control aspects of your experience, to make choices based on your preferences, and to give consent. Understanding what you can control, the choices you'll need to make, and what it means to consent to or refuse treatment are tools I think all pregnant people can benefit from.

- **Control** *is the power to influence or direct behavior and the course of events. It is the exercise of authoritative influence.*

In childbirth, there are things we can control in advance, like selecting a birth location and care provider, and there are things that might be unpredictable, like your water breaking before labor or going into labor before your planned Cesarean birth. Your labor might be faster or slower than imagined. It might be so much more difficult or so much less difficult than you prepared for. You might be planning a vaginal birth but find yourself in an operating room for a Cesarean birth. Birth is unpredictable, and this can feel out of control.

Speaking about her fears for her birth, Erika told me, "In my normal life, I am kind of a control freak. I think what scares me the most about birth is the idea that I have no control at all." This is a sentiment I've heard repeatedly. The unpredictability and vulnerability of birth can be frightening, and the possibility of being out of control can feel uncomfortable and unsafe. Being in a clinical setting heightens this for some, especially imagining needing emergency treatment.

In birth there are many ways you can remain in control and retain the feeling of having control, even in the face of plans changing or surprises. A sense of control can be regained by making plans (for aspects that can be planned), through making choices when available, and through your emotional reaction to your experiences. I've helped hundreds of people navigate moments where their plans needed to change—an induction of labor being recommended, a Cesarean birth becoming necessary, a care provider that's no longer available, a partner who can't be present, a test result that makes an epidural no longer a safe option, a baby coming earlier than anticipated. I remind people that even as things are changing in ways they might not like or that might feel out of control, this is still their birth experience and they can still work to make it a positive experience, where they feel as in control as possible.

What it means to have control (or feel out of control) varies from person to person. It might mean feeling like you have all the information needed or that you are treated well. It might mean that you are given a meaningful say in what's happening to you and are able to make decisions. It might mean that you feel safe, that your privacy is respected, or your modesty is not compromised. These feelings of being "in control" are partially about negotiating what can be controlled, but they're also about having choices and being able to give consent.

- ***Choice*** *is the act of selecting. It's making a decision when faced with two or more possibilities or paths forward.*

In planning for your birth you'll need to make choices about where you'll give birth, who you'd like with you, and what type of experience you'd like. You'll be able to weigh the policies and practices of different locations and providers, and make choices about what matches your desires. You'll make choices about having your partner, friends, family, or a doula with you for support. In labor, you can make choices about smaller things, like the music playing or what you're wearing, and about bigger things like receiving a medication or a medical procedure.

Often people describe their birth as a series of things that happened to them rather than choices they made. This might sound like simple semantics, but it's an important distinction. For example, the choice to have pain medication, such as an epidural, is often described as either an inability or failure ("I couldn't do it" or "It was impossible" or "I caved and asked for drugs") rather than a rational choice made by someone with a preference ("I decided I wanted pain relief"). Similarly, many describe a Cesarean birth as something that happened to them and not as part of their own decision-making. While there are rare emergencies, almost all Cesareans are the result of a conversation between a provider and a patient where you are asked to weigh your care provider's opinion about what is happening and the pros and cons of giving birth via a Cesarean before consenting.

I believe it's more powerful and positive to have made a choice rather than to have felt backed up against a wall, out of options, or incapable. I encourage my clients, and you, to own your decisions and honor the choices you make, whatever they are. Make a choice to have pain medication or skip it. Make a decision to have a Cesarean if that feels like it's become the safest or most desirable option. You have choices, and I encourage you to make decisions in your birth without apology.

- *Consent is the act of giving permission for something to happen. It's agreeing with and authorizing a plan of action.*

Consent is such an essential concept in birth, and in all medical care, but it's often glossed over. In all clinical settings, a care provider should get informed consent for any care they provide. In practice this might translate to a thoughtful conversation about the pros and cons of the care being offered or the test being recommended, but often it translates to having someone sign a piece of paper they haven't read or understood. This is not really informed consent.

In order for you to give permission, you need to understand why something is being suggested. What are the pros and cons? What are the risks and benefits? What alternatives exist? Discussing the options, taking time (when possible) to make a decision, and then consenting with full knowledge helps you feel in control of the experience.

Further, part of the consent process is the option of what's called "informed refusal." If informed consent is understanding the treatment recommended and consenting, informed refusal is also understanding the recommendation but declining. In birth, this might mean, for example, that your provider routinely recommends everyone be induced by their due date, but you decline induction, waiting for labor to begin spontaneously. It might mean your birth location has a policy against laboring people eating or drinking, but you opt to stay hydrated orally. You might be someone who has a religious objection to a blood transfusion, even in a life-threatening situation, and you have the right to refuse. You're not obligated to consent to recommendations from your providers—it's your choice when you consent or refuse treatment.

Pregnancy and childbirth can be particularly vulnerable times to navigate your choices because the decisions you make for yourself are influenced by your sense of what might be best for your baby. So often pregnant people say to me that they're open to whatever actually needs to happen clinically but that they don't want the fear of something bad happening to their baby used to manipulate them into unnecessary interventions or rushed decisions. This is a challenge and an excellent reason to be thoughtful in selecting a provider and birth team so you surround yourself with people who know what your preferences are and work with you to make sure you're able to make informed choices.

Throughout this book, the information, tips, worksheets, and stories are meant to help you negotiate the three Cs. A positive birth is one where you have control of the controllable elements, access to real and meaningful choices, clear information, nonjudgmental support, and informed consent (or refusal). That's a positive birth, whatever that looks like for you.

READING YOUR BIRTH PLAN

I remind my clients often that I don't care what choices they make. It doesn't matter to me where they give birth, if they hire a doctor or a midwife, who they have at their birth, what they consent to or refuse. I don't do this work to sway people toward specific choices but rather, to make sure you have all the information, support, and space needed to make the choices. I don't care about the specifics of those choices. So many people in our lives, especially in pregnancy and parenting, have opinions about what we should do or how to do it. I don't want to offer you opinions. I want to give you information and options to make your own decisions.

This book is organized loosely around the order in which the information might be most useful for you. For most people, making a plan about where you'd like to give birth is the first choice you might need to make. As such, the first section offers an overview of your birthing options and why location matters with chapters on hospitals, birth centers, and homebirth. Each chapter details what's available in each location, risks and benefits, reasons this location might appeal (or be a bad option) for your needs, and information you might want to gather about the specific birth options in your area.

After you have a clear sense of where you'd like to give birth and what your options are, the next decision most people make is selecting a care provider and thinking about birth support. The second section is organized around the birth team you'll build, including picking a doctor or midwife, hiring a doula (or not), and support from a partner, friends, or family. This section begins with an overview on building a birth team and then has chapters specifically about doctors, midwives, and doulas. I detail the different types of doctors who assist with birth, as well as variation in how midwives are trained and licensed and what this might mean for you. I discuss how the model of care might vary between providers and offer the pros and cons of working with different types of providers, as well as working with a doula.

Following this, there's a section on labor and birth starting with a long chapter about labor that details what's happening in your body. This chapter is meant to help you know what's probable and possible, how to interpret the signs or symptoms you experience, and how labor progresses (both clinically and what you might experience). This chapter includes information on your baby dropping, the mucus plug, water breaking, contractions, bleeding, shaking, throwing up, rectal pressure, pushing, your placenta, the first hour after birth, and more.

The next chapter is on common interventions during labor and childbirth. This chapter will help you understand what a provider might be looking for if they ask for a urine sample, how fetal monitoring works, what it means to have your water broken, what Group Beta Strep is, how epidurals and narcotics work to help with pain, what an assisted vaginal delivery is, what an episiotomy is, and more. Many of these things might be routine in your location, like fetal monitoring or IV access, but you'll have choices about what you consent to or refuse. This chapter is intended to help you make informed choices.

The final chapter in this section is on thinking through your preferences, making plans for your birth, labor-coping strategies, and how plans can change in pregnancy or labor.

The fourth section is a series of chapters on specific childbirth situations you might be planning for (or might end up in if plans change). The first chapter is on induction of labor, navigating your choices during an induction, and situations where you might consider refusing an induction. Nearly a quarter of births are induced,[1] so this chapter might be helpful to read through regardless of your plans. Next is a chapter on planning a vaginal birth after Cesarean birth (VBAC). If you've already had a Cesarean birth, this chapter can help you think through whether having another Cesarean birth or a vaginal birth is your preference. The third chapter in this section is on giving birth to twins or multiples, and will be helpful if you're navigating how your options change when giving birth to more than one baby. This section ends with a chapter on planning for a Cesarean birth, including choices about seeing and holding your baby, and making the operating room a more familiar or welcoming space if you'd like.

Throughout the book there are interview guides, lists, tips, and worksheets to help you pick a birth location, find a provider or a doula, pack your bag, think about your preferences, make a birth plan, turn a breech baby, plan a Cesarean, navigate the NICU (neonatal intensive care unit), chest/breastfeed, and care for yourself. These are tools you can use as you navigate your options and choices. You will also find birth stories (all generously shared with permission) and quotes from new parents about their experiences in every chapter.

Throughout this book, and throughout your pregnancy, you will hear and read the term "risk" many times, a reflection of how common this term is in obstetrics. Pregnancies are categorized as high risk and low risk. Behavior and choices might be described as risky. A provider might tell you about the risk of various complications or the risks associated with different interventions. Risk means exposure to danger, harm, or loss, and in pregnancy, this term can feel scary and highlight the vulnerability of being pregnant. I have used this language of risk throughout the book, mirroring the language of obstetrics, but I want to acknowledge how challenging this word can be for some people up front and hopefully soften its impact as you read on. In my practice, I try to spend more time with clients thinking about probability and possibility, because it can remind us that while something is possible (that a risk exists), it is most often not very probable. As you read on, please keep this in mind.

When you're reading this book, you might also notice that the language throughout is gender inclusive: I use terms like pregnant people, parent, chest/breastfeeding. For some, this might be new and could feel awkward or confusing; for others it might be welcome. I've read critiques of this inclusion. Some have argued that using inclusive language feels like a type of erasure or removal of women from birth, but not everyone who gives birth identifies as a woman—that's a fact and it should not be ignored. When I'm speaking broadly about pregnancy, birth, or parenthood, I've used inclusive terms to open space for all pregnant people and families. When I am speaking about a specific person and their experience, or quoting someone, I have used the language they use to identify themselves.

You might also notice several places where I specifically address recommendations given to pregnant people based on body size. This is important to me as an advocate for birthing people of all sizes, as a body positive activist and author, and as a fat woman (a term I self-identify with, not an insult the way "fat" is often used). I was given advice during my pregnancies based not on my health but on my size, and I've seen this repeatedly with clients. I worry about how a provider's bias and beliefs about bodies impacts medical advice in ways not medically supported. I worry about people being overtreated, such as the increase in routine inductions and Cesareans recommended for larger pregnant people.[2] I also worry about how this impacts thin people, as I've seen thin clients instructed to ignore bad test results (like gestational diabetes) because of their size and presumed health. We must do better than this.

You might similarly notice several places where I've noted that providers or medical organizations cite different risks or outcomes based on race. I've noted that this shouldn't be seen as a reflection of biological difference but rather as the result of racism. Recent media attention continues to expose the profound disparities in outcomes for pregnant people of color.[3] The media has forced the beginning of a long overdue national dialogue on racism in our health care systems, and politicians and policy makers are pushing new programs in an effort to improve care and outcomes.[4] Yet even with more widespread acknowledgment of the problem, providers will still, for example, use a VBAC calculator (a data tool for assessing the likelihood of a successful vaginal birth after a Cesarean) result to discourage a person of color from having a vaginal birth without seemingly even recognizing they're furthering the problem (see chapter 12). If you are a pregnant person of color, understanding how racism is impacting your care might be important to ensure you have the safest experience possible.

Finally, I want to note more broadly that we all bring our bodies to the experience of giving birth. That means we bring our actual bodies and also our histories of bodies. This might mean you bring a history of feeling strong and capable, healthy, or safe in your body. It might mean you bring a history of disease, disability, or difference. It might mean your experience of your body has been mediated by bias, prejudice, or privilege. It might mean you bring a history of abuse and surviving, birth loss or reproductive trauma, or feeling pleasure or pain (or both). How you navigate your choices and what control and consent mean for you might be influenced by your body history. Give yourself space to have the experience you want or need.

My hope is that all the information and tools I've provided might make it easier for you to pick where, with whom, and in what way *you* would like to give birth. Throughout, I've tried to highlight what's possible or probable with the aim of quelling anxieties, dispelling myths, and sharing information. My aim is to inspire you to feel confident in yourself and in your birth team, to mobilize informed decision-making, and ultimately to help you have a birth where you're treated well and feel positive about your experience. I've showcased the widest range of options, experiences, families, and decisions wherever possible. While some information could be hard to read—especially if descriptions of medical tools or interventions are tough for you—my hope is also that you're reminded throughout that birth, in all the forms it takes, can be beautiful, powerful, and good.

I

WHERE SHOULD I GIVE BIRTH?

1

CHOOSING YOUR BIRTH LOCATION

My phone rang in the middle of the night, not an uncommon or particularly noteworthy experience given my work. My brother's name appeared on the screen. I answered, wondering if the call was a mistake. Sean's worried voice confirmed it wasn't a mistake. His wife, Shail, was seven months pregnant, planning a homebirth, but her water had just broken too early.

Shail's an organic farmer—she raises grass-fed animals for meat—and is one of the most disciplined people I know. She uses no chemical cleaners, wears organic clothing, buys only local food, and uses zero plastic (not even organic cheese sold in plastic wrap). Shail approached her pregnancy with similarly strong convictions: she hired midwives for prenatal care and wanted no medications, no interventions, and no testing, including ultrasounds, unless necessary.

After her water broke, that plan changed rapidly. At the hospital, they did an ultrasound to measure the amniotic fluid and check the size and position of the baby. Having no ultrasounds at nearly thirty-three weeks pregnant is almost unheard of. The sonographer spread cold gel on her belly, and a grainy image came onto the screen. The technician showed them "baby A" in a frank breech in the birth canal (his butt down) and "baby B" above him, sideways. Surprise twins are a rarity in the age of ultrasound, but my niece and nephew shocked us all.

With her cervix rapidly opening and her baby in a breech position, a Cesarean birth was planned, but the hospital lacked the appropriate technology to support two premature babies. She was in active labor, so they transported her by ambulance to a larger hospital in a nearby town. Adjusting to the change of location, unknown doctors, potential health complications for the babies, a

Cesarean birth, and suddenly being the parents of *two* babies was overwhelming. Born just under and over four pounds, respectively, Tule and Slate were healthy and robust for their gestational age but needed nurses, doctors, and the neonatal intensive care unit (NICU). Machines helped them breathe, as well as monitored their heart rates, temperature, and respiration; and they were fed through IV, a feeding tube, and then a bottle before nursing. After a few weeks, they were big enough to go home, where they've thrived.

When my phone rang that night, it wasn't my brother I was expecting to hear from. I had a client in the neighborhood, Ana, who was well past her due date, expecting her second son. I was sure the call was from her. She was, like Shail, planning a homebirth. She'd planned to have her first in a birth center but transferred to a hospital ultimately. This time Ana wanted a homebirth, but she needed to go into labor soon or she'd have to transfer again. She'd been told various techniques to get labor started, but no amount of acupuncture, sex, walking, or spicy food had made the baby come. Thankfully, a couple of days after Shail gave birth, on a sunny June afternoon, Ana's son was born at home.

Just days apart, these two births are a contrast between what we plan for and what happens, of what we want and need, of the difference between the comforts of home and the technologies of the hospital, but mostly the contrast in how we're treated. Ana's birth, in a pool in her kitchen, was the birth Shail had planned for. Shail was disappointed by her experience. The staff were not kind. I suspect they judged and blamed her, thought she was foolish for refusing an ultrasound. They didn't understand how she could be unhappy even while understanding the need for the interventions. Ana was elated. She felt loved and supported while she met her baby surrounded by spices, pots and pans, and a giant bowl of watermelon.

I don't present these births as a tool for endorsing homebirth. My niece and nephew are likely alive because they were born in a hospital. I share these stories as a tool for thinking about the importance of how we plan both for the birth we want and the unpredictability of birth. For Shail, there wasn't a good backup plan—just a midwife who ultimately wasn't there. When her water broke, all her plans vanished. They were two shell-shocked parents reeling from a transfer. I ached for being far away when they needed more guidance, compassion, and familiar faces.

For Ana, she'd already faced a transfer from a birth center to a hospital with her first and understood this possibility as she planned her second birth. Her first birth was a positive experience because she planned for the possibility of a transfer and brought support with her. With her second birth, Ana planned for a transfer if needed but had the experience she hoped for (as did Shail when she gave birth at home six years later).

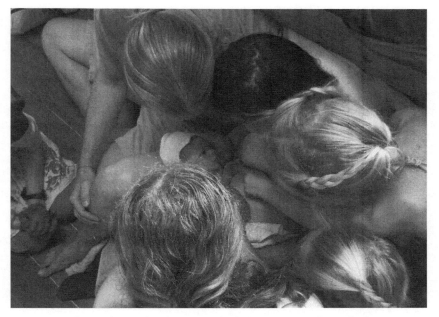

Left to right: My brother Sean, Shail, their twins, and a midwife.

Picking a place to give birth—home, a birth center, a hospital—is an important decision and one that's often not given much thought. It's not uncommon to continue care with an obstetrician (OB) or midwife you've seen for routine well care, or to select a new provider with little thought to the institution that provider is connected with. Yet location is enormously important in planning for a positive birth. The policies and practices, philosophy and approach, and, as Shail's birth demonstrates, sometimes the technologies and physicians available, are important.

There's no one right place to have a baby—the key is to figure out what's important to you. Picking a location that reflects your values and beliefs, matches your health and clinical needs, resonates with your sense of safety and support, and ideally, that includes thought-out contingency plans, is central to having a positive birth experience.

Depending on your location and resources, the options available to you might be quite large or quite small. You might have dozens of hospitals to pick from or just one that's near enough. A birth center might be available nearby, or not. State laws about homebirth and midwives might further constrain your options. Insurance coverage might limit who you can see. And, of course, there are your preferences. In each of the chapters that follow, there's lots of information and tools to help you find the right birth location.

Nearly eight years after Shail gave birth, on a chilly Thursday night, I met a new potential client in a Brooklyn cafe. Unlike most meet-and-greets, Neta said she was already convinced she wanted me as her doula and signed the agreement immediately. The conversation she wanted to have was about where she should give birth. Only a few weeks pregnant, Neta was already overwhelmed. She had Medicaid for insurance, which she feared would overly constrain her choices. The information she'd gathered from friends and the internet was not helping.

Even with Medicaid, the options available for Neta actually included a dozen hospitals with varied policies and practices, at least one birth center, and a list of homebirth midwives. She had lots of options, more than many people in other areas. I still couldn't tell her which place was the right place, but I helped Neta sort through the options by asking her a series of questions about what was most important to her and what her "best-case scenario" looked like. We talked through her hopes and fears, the stories she'd heard, and her questions, such as:

> *Will the hospital require me to stay in the bed the whole time I'm laboring?*
> *Can you give birth in a hospital without getting an epidural? Could you help me do that?*
> *Who'd be part of my care in a hospital besides my doctor or midwife? Can I control this?*
> *Will I have to have male care providers, or can I insist on women only?*
> *Will they take my baby away? Do they do tests on them away from me after the birth?*
> *If I birth outside of a hospital, who takes care of these things for the baby?*
> *Do I have too small of an apartment for a homebirth?*
> *What about our cats? Can you give birth with them in the house?*
> *Is it crazy to give birth at home—what if something bad happens?*
> *What if I change my mind during a homebirth and want to go to the hospital?*
> *What if I plan a homebirth and need to be in the hospital for a medical reason?*
> *Is an out-of-hospital birth center a middle ground between a homebirth and the hospital?*
> *What about a birth center inside a hospital? How does that work?*
> *Do all of these places take insurance, or do I have to pay for it myself?*

Long before talking about individual doctors or midwives Neta might work with, we hashed out birth location options. Within each location there were providers she could interview and choose from, but before that she needed to imagine the birth she wanted and where that would be. Her questions reflected her preferences and led to the choices she made. You'll have different questions, plans, preferences, needs, and options available to you.

When I spoke with Lina and Annie about how they picked where to give birth, they both described experiences with their mothers that impacted where they felt most safe and supported for birth. Lina described her decision to give birth in a hospital with an OB, saying:

> I grew up in New York City with a single mother, and once when I was about nine I had to call 911 and travel by ambulance to a hospital with my mother who was suffering from a debilitating migraine. Showing the paramedics into my mother's bedroom and watching them strap her to the stretcher and roll her out of our building lobby, out onto the busy sidewalk full of people, and into the ambulance was frightening and stressful. I knew that I probably wouldn't do well attempting a homebirth with the fear of that potential experience lodged in my mind.

For Annie, her experiences being in the hospital with her mother during cancer treatments had a different impact on her decision-making. She wrote:

> I was too afraid to go to the hospital. I had spent the past four months in and out of the hospital, the nursing home, and Urgent Care. I saw how they worked. I saw my mom push her buzzer to summon the nurse and I watched the second hand tick around the clock until she got a response. No way was I doing that if I could help it. I hated the hospital and suspected that I would feel helpless and disempowered there. I knew I didn't want any unnecessary interventions or pain medication, and felt like I would be bullied or tempted in a hospital setting.
>
> I had several friends who had given birth at home, and I think this helped me feel like it was more normal than it actually is. I wanted to feel supported and empowered. I did not want to be talked down to or treated like I was not the one who was fully in charge. I did not want to be condescended to. Perhaps I was being a control freak? Maybe I also like the political implications of saying "fuck you" to the establishment? Either way, I wanted to be with people who believed that birth was normal. This is hugely important to me.

The right place for each of them to give birth was different, but they both had positive experiences. In what follows, I discuss all birth locations in greater detail with descriptions. Each chapter includes information about the providers and technologies available (and the variability of that) plus the reasons that location might appeal to you.

2

GIVING BIRTH
IN A HOSPITAL

On a cold winter night, I took a cab through near-empty Brooklyn streets. I'd been texting with Tara and Juan for hours about the progress of labor. Things were getting stronger, and Tara asked me to head over to their house. She was laboring in her bedroom with dim lights and a radiator working overtime, making the room hot and dry. Between contractions she curled up on her bed and seemed to fall asleep for a minute. When the contraction returned, Tara jumped up, threw off the blanket, and held Juan as she moaned and swayed. As quickly as it came, it passed and she silently moved back to the bed in a sleep-like state.

There was no talking in the room, but an eclectic mix of music was streamed through the TV. Biggie's voice came through the speakers. The track begins with a dedication: to the teachers who said he wouldn't amount to anything, the people who called the police when he was trying to feed his daughter by dealing, and all the people in the struggle. This dedication is familiar to me—Biggie is a Brooklyn icon—but the song is best known for a phrase in the second verse: "Spread love, it's the Brooklyn way." Perfect for a birth, where oxytocin, a love hormone, brings on contractions. I smiled to myself as Tara jumped up for another contraction.

As the sun came up, we headed to the hospital. Tara was nearly fully dilated, in the heart of transitioning to pushing her baby out. She preferred the floor to the bed, so we laid absorbent pads under and around her. Her doctor came in and out periodically to check in, help fix the monitors, and remind Tara he was available. When Tara began pushing with contractions, she moved to the bed on her hands and knees. Shortly after, her son slid into the world and was placed on her chest. His umbilical cord pulsed blood for the next few minutes as Juan and Tara explored their new baby. While they'd considered birthing elsewhere, the hospital appealed the most, and they were thrilled to have a low-intervention experience with the added security of interventions nearby if needed.

Tara and Juan's choice to birth in a hospital is the same as the vast majority of people giving birth in the US today. Though this wasn't always the case—homebirth in this country used to be common—giving birth in the hospital has been the norm since the 1940s. Nearly four million babies are born annually in the US, and more than 98 percent are born inside hospitals.[1] The 2 percent of babies not born in hospitals are either people who accidentally gave birth before arriving at the hospital or people who planned out-of-hospital birth center or homebirths.

Hospitals are the most accessible of the options: everyone can give birth in a hospital. You'll read that for birth centers and homebirths, screening by care providers to ensure you're healthy and having a fairly low-risk pregnancy is required. People with a variety of risk factors are disqualified from birthing outside of hospitals, but hospitals do not routinely disqualify anyone (with the exception of cases where an individual hospital doesn't have the appropriate technologies or doctors to treat you or your baby and needs to transfer you to another hospital).

For most people, hospitals are the place they feel safest giving birth, regardless of any known need for the technologies and clinical capacities hospitals have available. Hospitals can offer a sense of security. With several generations now born predominantly inside of hospitals, this option often feels most familiar, responsible, and practical.

WHAT HOSPITALS HAVE TO OFFER

There are a lot of things available in hospitals not available in any other birth location. Hospitals offer access to pain medication, such as epidurals, and have anesthesia teams available. If needed, they have operating rooms and teams of doctors and nurses prepared to perform surgery. They have pediatricians on staff to help treat babies after they're born. NICUs are available in many (but not all) hospitals. Hospitals are also required by law to provide at least a forty-eight-hour stay after a vaginal birth and at least a ninety-six-hour stay after a Cesarean birth.[2] While you can choose to leave earlier, this opportunity to heal, learn to chest/breastfeed, and begin parenting in an environment with staff available full-time might be comforting.

Some of us have personal memories or cultural references (TV, movies) that have led us to think of hospitals as overcrowded, undesirable, or impersonal, but many of my clients remark that the hospital is more warm, pleasant, and accommodating than they imagined.

When I was pregnant the first time, my husband's grandmother described her births to me. She recalled checking in to the hospital on an assigned day but couldn't remember anything else that happened for nearly a week. She did that four times. A medication combo called "twilight sleep" was likely given to her along with Pitocin (a synthetic form of the hormone oxytocin, which causes contractions). Rather than pushing, she had episiotomies (a cut to her perineum) and forceps were used to pull her babies out vaginally. She was awake through this, but the morphine in the twilight sleep mixture reduced her pain while scopolamine made her amnesic. She didn't have negative feelings about her experiences, but they didn't sound good to me. The loss of control, absence of consent, and abandonment of choice were not what I wanted.

When my mother was pregnant with me, she lived thirty minutes outside of Madison, Wisconsin, and wanted to give birth in the hospital where she'd birthed my brother. That said, she didn't want a repeat of her last experience. She wrote a letter to administrators of the hospital laying out her concerns and requests for her upcoming birth. In her letter—a handwritten note I found a copy of when helping her move to California years ago—she described her first birth in 1971 as "endless tubes and IVs" in a crowded hospital where she was left to labor "in the hallway behind a screen" with "noise and confusion in an overheated ward." She wrote: "Women were shifted up and down the hall, room to room and bed to bed and I wandered through the hall holding my IV and watching six babies being born." It was a "large social gathering" with staff everywhere offering unnecessary "opinions and conjecture on everything from the screamer down the hall with the epidural to the loud drunk whose wife was having a Cesarean."

Her next birth in 1976 was a better experience. Her doctor was great—he "adjusted the table to a sitting position, lowered the lights and joked about the noisy air compressor playing contemporary jazz." My father held her hand as she birthed with "no episiotomy, no mess and no fuss. We were all laughing. . . . I liked being able to hold my babe before the cord was cut and not having him rushed off to the nursery for several hours. It was pleasant."

Yet, my mom reflected in her letter on the places where they could have done better: she had to wait outside while in labor because the door was locked, there were "about eight nurses with nothing to do," she was made to switch beds five times during an hour of labor and one night of recovery, and someone "got sloppy" with silver nitrate (no longer routinely used) and burned my brother. She wrote, "It was still a much nicer way to have a baby . . . but there is another way that could be even nicer." Her requests for my birth: one nurse, one bed, one room (ideally with a washroom and a window), the baby not taken to the nursery, and "privacy would be a pleasure." My mom wrote: "It may be another brief labor and delivery and I would like to enjoy it rather than being awed by all the activity around me."

On a hot July night, my mom arrived at the hospital far into her labor and gave birth shortly after in the asked-for private labor room. She stayed only half a day and took me home without any separation. I asked her about my birth recently, and she said no one had ever asked the hospital for these accommodations. They allowed them for her, but they did not change their practice for others. Her total bill came to $38—the fee for a half day in the room. My father is frugal to a fault, and I've joked much of my life that I'm his favorite child (apologies to my brothers) because I was a good deal from the beginning. At less than $40, my birth was *on sale!*

The common protocols and practices in most hospitals have changed dramatically for the better since our grandmothers and mothers gave birth. Much of what my mom requested for her birth is now readily available. The environment tends to be warm, supportive, and welcoming. My clients often exclaim with enthusiasm how much nicer the birthing rooms are than they had imagined. Unfortunately, there still are hospitals with tiny rooms and older facilities than people had hoped for—a good reason to do your homework when selecting your birth location—but many have spacious rooms with comfortable couches and chairs, bathrooms with showers or tubs, and speakers for music. The staff and nurses are usually friendly and kind, expressing interest in your birth preferences and helping advocate for your preferences whenever possible.

Most people birthing in hospitals can have at least two support people throughout labor and delivery. Doulas are usually welcomed and encouraged (or at least tolerated). A support person can also be present in the operating room in the event that a Cesarean birth is needed. Some hospitals will also allow you to have your other children with you (although some ban kids from the birthing rooms, so this is good to confirm if it's important to you).

Some hospitals have wireless monitoring available for more mobility (otherwise fetal monitoring limits movement to about three feet). Some hospitals also provide low-tech labor aids commonly found in birth centers such as yoga balls, peanut balls, squat bars, and birthing stools (all can help with labor and vaginal birth).

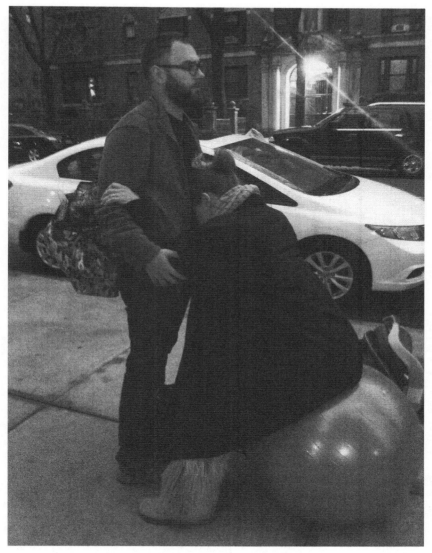

Laboring on a yoga ball while waiting for the cab.

There are usually private rooms to labor and birth in, and often private rooms are available postpartum as well. Many hospitals are moving away from mandatory nursery stays and opting instead to keep healthy babies with their parents (unless you request a break). Many nurses have extensive training in chest/breastfeeding and newborn care and can help new parents as they begin their journey.

In imagining your hospital birth, it's important to find answers to questions you might have about the following: policies and practices about support people or kids in birthing rooms; rules about eating or drinking in labor; requirements for fetal monitoring; IV access; mandatory nursery stays; your access to showers and tubs or labor aids like balls; the overall rate of interventions and Cesarean births; access to privacy in birth and afterward; and support for postpartum preferences that might be important to you, such as chest/breastfeeding, access to a nursery, the policy on bathing babies, and more. You'll also want to look into practical questions about proximity and expected travel time, insurance coverage (because $38 is no longer the going rate), and the specific doctors or midwives you'll have access to.

POSITIVE, AFFIRMING, SUPPORTED HOSPITAL BIRTHS

As I was writing this, I was waiting on the arrival of a baby I expected would be born any day. Over a week past her due date, Linda shared with me that she worried she was keeping the baby in. She loved being pregnant so much—it was a magical experience for her and one she was perhaps not entirely ready to give up. We talked about it, about what came next, and about the process of letting go to get ready for labor. A few days later Linda felt small twinges of the labor brewing. By the evening those twinges became contractions, and as it got dark, she was actively breathing and working through contractions. She labored through the night, pacing and lunging and squatting and breathing in the too narrow hallways of her tiny West Village apartment. It felt good for her to move through the contractions. The lunging and squatting felt like they helped the baby come. Labor continued, and early in the morning, we took a cab to the hospital. Linda's obstetrician met us there. He's a gentle man with a soft voice who apologizes often and is quick to remind his clients that his recommendations are suggestions but they ultimately have all the decision-making power.

Linda moved from the toilet to the bed to her husband's arms, and back again. She paced the hospital room like she'd paced her apartment. Her husband had a steady soundtrack of classics from the sixties and seventies and contemporary folk music playing. Doris Day's voice filled the room singing "Dream a Little Dream of Me," a song she'd sung in college, and she began to sing while perched on the edge of the bed. A contraction came, and she sang through it, commenting afterward that she found the singing to be helpful. A few hours later, she was lying on her side with a peanut ball between her legs (peanut balls are a type of physical therapy ball often used in labor to hold your legs while lying down). Linda began to cry. These were not tears of sadness but of letting go. Looking into her husband's eyes, their faces a few inches apart, she was sobbing. I was sitting on the other side of the bed, massaging her lower back and butt to help her stay on the bed and rest her legs.

John Lennon's voice came through the speakers, and she started to sing "Imagine" through her tears. Her husband joined in, and I followed shortly after. After hundreds of births, it was the first time I sang with a client. As we sang, her doctor entered the room. I wondered what he thought as he took in the scene. As doulas, our relationships with clinical care providers and staff can be a bit surveilled. Are we following the rules? Being helpful enough to warrant our presence? When the chorus returned, her doctor joined us in song.

Sometimes people fear hospital births will be too clinical, too cold, too impersonal, or too predetermined by rules and policies and protocols. You might fear that obstetricians, trained as surgeons, will be quick to recommend clinical interventions or unwanted medications (and some likely are). You might be concerned that a doctor could be ill prepared to support you through a labor and birth that doesn't require their surgical skills. You might worry that hospital-based midwives are too clinical or lack enough power to fully support you. What if you just need patience and time? It's true that sometimes births are expedited by interventions in hospitals. Sometimes a more patient approach might net a different result. With Cesarean birthrates more than 50 percent in some hospitals, this is certainly worth paying attention to.[3] But I want to also caution you not to be too quick to stereotype hospital births or the people who choose them.

A professor and accomplished author, my friend Marilyn is one of the smartest, fiercest people I know, and when she agreed to send me her birth stories, I was fascinated to read them. I was also disappointed, although not surprised, to read that she was made to feel she was failing in her births. She and her girlfriend planned a homebirth in San Francisco with their first daughter. After laboring all night she was in so much pain and she felt she couldn't go on any longer. She knew that changing her plans and heading to the hospital would be seen as failure to her midwives. Her friend saw through her anxiety and physical turmoil and said, "If you want to go to the hospital, I'll take you there." She nodded, and they drove to the hospital. Marilyn recalled feeling guilty when she said yes to the epidural but proud when they wheeled her down the hall with her baby on her chest, saying to her mother, "Isn't she beautiful?"

All three of Marilyn's daughters were born in hospitals—her first birth was a homebirth transfer in San Francisco, her second daughter arrived so quickly at a Brooklyn hospital that her doctor didn't make it, and her third daughter, after Marilyn's trauma of multiple miscarriages and a termination for a trisomy pregnancy, was born in a Manhattan hospital with a high-risk obstetrician. In conversation with me, Marilyn recalled a moment when she spoke with another feminist scholar, one who has focused on childbirth and midwifery care throughout her academic career. The colleague made her feel like she had been "duped" for giving birth in hospitals, for having pain medication, and for working with doctors. Marilyn's standing as a feminist was questioned because of her birthing choices.

In talking about the hospital births of her two children, Zoe told me, "I know some people think hospitals are the enemy of beautiful births," but she felt "wonderfully cared for and supported the entire time." She acknowledged that other people really struggle after unwanted Cesarean births (or other changes in birth plans) but said that her doctors, nurses, and doula were all "knowledgeable, professional, patient," and this helped her feel really positive about both of her births—a Cesarean birth and a vaginal birth after a Cesarean (VBAC). Similarly, Brie described her hospital births as wonderful experiences, saying, "I know the hospital can be crowded or overwhelming, but we had a really awesome team: just my one doctor, just one nurse. They both helped me through the whole labor and it was perfect." Brie loved having access to an epidural and felt this helped enormously in making her birth experience positive. Nancy said

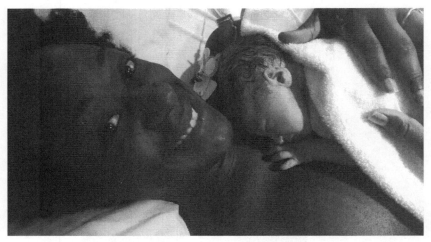

New mother holding newborn minutes after giving birth.

working with a midwife in a hospital was the perfect combination of "all the safety of the hospital with all the personalized care and support of a midwife." Nancy's midwife was supportive of her plan to get an epidural, and when a test result prompted an induction of labor shortly before her due date, her midwife's guidance through the whole process was so reassuring.

The wrong match with a care provider or a hospital with outdated or overly restrictive policies and practices can certainly lead to a disappointing experience. Ideally there are options, and you can work to avoid this type of experience. The moments I described above—Tara welcoming her son her way, Linda's birth team joining her in song, Marilyn choosing the hospital when others felt she should "know better," Zoe and Brie and Nancy feeling cared for and supported—are perfect reminders of what a hospital birth experience can be. Positive, affirming, supported births can happen in every birth setting.

3

GIVING BIRTH IN A BIRTH CENTER

On a warm spring morning, just barely light out, I walked a few short blocks from my home to Susan, who'd started contracting during the night. We'd exchanged texts for several hours, and she was ready for me to join her. Susan loved the water to help her cope with the contractions, and I found her in the shower—her bathroom steamy with a nest of towels and pillows on the floor. For the next several hours she worked through strong contractions with lots of massage, movement, and encouragement from her husband and me. She labored at home until contractions were really intense—nearly unbearable—before calling a cab and driving together over the Manhattan Bridge to the in-hospital birth center where her midwife was waiting.

When we arrived at the hospital, we were ushered into a large room with several curtained-off hospital beds, IV poles, fetal monitoring machines, and shelves of medical supplies. She was just beginning to feel the urge to push, and her midwife's exam showed she was fully dilated. The birth center Susan gave birth in requires all patients go through triage before getting access to the birth center. This triage step aims to ensure that only healthy, low-risk people with no labor complications are admitted into the birth center. Susan had all the required things: twenty minutes of fetal monitoring, a normal blood pressure reading, a normal temperature, a blood draw, a catheter placed in her arm for emergency IV access, and an internal examination of her cervix by her midwife. A whole lot of strong back massage made it possible for Susan to stay in the bed during this, but she was counting down the minutes until she could get up again. Finished with triage, we walked to the birth center together. Her husband was on one side of her, the midwife on the other side, and me trailing behind, with bags and a camera.

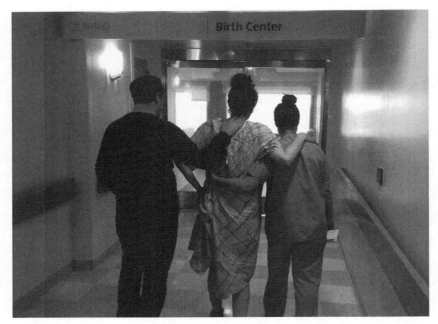

Walking to the birth center.

Inside the birth center there was a large Jacuzzi tub we started filling. The water was loud so Susan retreated to the bathroom and opted for the immediacy of a shower. She moved from the shower to the tub when it was filled. Susan was focused and determined, hardly speaking. She used the space between contractions to rest. Finally, as the pressure to push grew stronger, she moved to the queen-sized bed in the center of the room, remaining on her hands and knees.

As the pressure during contractions grew, Susan moved from her hands and knees into something closer to kneeling while pushing. This worked well for her, but it didn't leave much space for the midwife behind her to reach the baby. The midwife was happy to sit on the bed behind her and reach through her legs to deliver the baby but needed Susan to stay more on her hands and knees, with her butt up rather than pushed into the bed. In order for her to do this during the final contractions, I sat in front of Susan and suggested she rest her forehead on my forehead, leaning forward into me. This helped her feel grounded and stable while also giving the midwife enough space. For me, it meant I was forehead to forehead with Susan as she pushed her baby out. I could feel the power of her pushes on my brow.

After her son was born, Susan moved into a reclined position with him on her chest skin to skin. With the help of her midwife, she delivered her placenta and was checked for any vaginal tears that might require stitches. We gave her something to drink and offered her snacks. Susan's husband snuggled in next to her on the big bed, both of them admiring and touching their newborn. Her baby started to show interest in feeding, and within an hour, he was nursing. That afternoon, they all headed back to Brooklyn to sleep in their own bed.

WHAT BIRTH CENTERS OFFER

Susan's birth is a perfect example of the promise of giving birth inside a birth center—a low-intervention, unmedicated birth with access to a tub, a larger bed, support for pushing and birthing in a variety of positions, and going home without a long hospital stay. Around the country, there are more than three hundred birth centers.[1] While Susan picked an in-hospital birth center, many birth centers in the US are freestanding. Currently, about 1 percent of births in the US take place inside birth centers, although that number is increasing.[2] Nearly half of the birth centers in the US were built in the last few years, and more are scheduled to open soon.[3] Birth centers cost about half the fees associated with the average hospital birth, and they're covered by most insurance plans.[4]

Birth centers are usually staffed by midwives, although occasionally obstetricians and family practice doctors work in birth centers. Because midwifery training and licensing varies (see chapter 6), birth centers are differently staffed and accredited. There are national guidelines for birth centers, but individual birth centers are not obligated to comply. State laws and local regulations vary significantly, and you should look into these as part of your decision-making around selecting a birth location.

Set up to offer an alternative to giving birth in a hospital, birth centers offer a homelike environment with nonhospital furniture such as larger beds, tubs for laboring or birthing, birthing stools, and sometimes ropes or slings from the ceiling to hold on to for supported squatting. The emphasis in birth centers is usually on normalizing birth and supporting unmedicated (or minimally medicated) and minimally interventionist experiences. Epidurals are not available in birth centers, although IV narcotics and inhaled nitrous oxide sometimes are.

Birth centers are typically equipped to monitor the vital signs of the laboring person and baby with blood pressure cuffs, thermometers, and fetal heart monitors. Interventions like IV hydration, antibiotic treatment, and breaking your water are usually available, while other interventions, such as induction of labor, assisted vaginal delivery, or treatment for conditions like preeclampsia or pregnancy-induced hypertension, are not typically supported in birth centers.

Eating and drinking during labor is not limited in birth centers. Family and other support people are welcomed, and pushing in any position the laboring person would like is encouraged (while more than 90 percent of people in hospitals birth lying down or in a semisitting position).[5] A newborn exam is provided either by a midwife or doctor so your baby never has to leave you. Early discharge is the norm: you might stay as little as a few hours or most of a day. Staying more than about eighteen hours is very rare for a birth center.

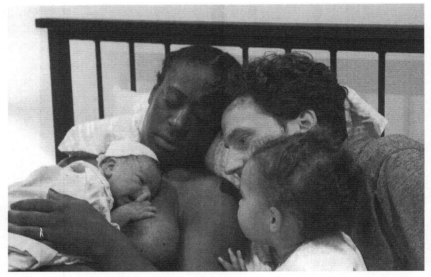

Enjoying the immediate postpartum in the homelike environment of a birth center.

There has been much research to support giving birth outside of hospitals—especially in birth centers—as not only safe, but at times even safer than giving birth on a hospital maternity floor. Because birth centers have more judicious use of intervention and medical technology while still being supported by skilled professionals, studies have shown that giving birth in a birth center decreases the likelihood of medical intervention without increasing risk,[6] a win-win situation if your pregnancy is low risk and you're interested in giving birth without an epidural.

WHO CAN GIVE BIRTH HERE? RISKING OUT
OF A BIRTH CENTER

Part of how birth centers create a safe environment is screening and monitoring to ensure their patients remain low risk. Many birth centers provide a list of conditions, complications, or circumstances that will result in you being "risked out" (often a stressful list to read). Each facility has its own list of what is "low risk" enough and what warrants being "risked out." Depending on the center, these criteria may be more (or less) evidence based.

There are some very clear conditions or complications that are generally agreed upon as reasons to not give birth in a birth center. These include prenatal problems with elevated blood pressure (and preeclampsia) or any health conditions that are incompatible with labor or a vaginal birth, problems with the placenta (such placenta previa), giving birth to twins or triplets, a prenatal diagnosis of a fetal condition that requires immediate pediatric or surgical care, or going into labor prematurely (usually before thirty-seven weeks). These are higher-risk conditions that warrant birthing in a hospital facility with obstetricians or maternal fetal medicine doctors, access to anesthesia and operating rooms, and a NICU with pediatricians.

Some birth centers also have specific requirements during the labor itself. For example, you might be required to be in active labor when you arrive (based on a cervical exam). This could mean laboring at home for much of your labor before going to the birth center. There might also be a requirement to transfer to a hospital if your water has been broken for a longer amount of time (such as eighteen or twenty-four hours). A transfer will also likely happen for signs of fetal distress, such as a high or low heart rate or meconium (baby poop) in your amniotic fluid.

There are higher-risk conditions that some birth centers will support. For example, some birth centers will risk you out for gestational diabetes, but others support people if their diabetes is well controlled. Similarly, being over thirty-five years old is considered higher risk (and labeled terribly as elderly or geriatric pregnancy), but many birth centers support people who are older than thirty-five years old (although most have some age cutoff). Additionally, having a vaginal birth after a Cesarean (VBAC) is considered higher risk and forces many people out of birth centers, but occasional birth centers do support VBACs. Also, the standard of care in the US is to recommend a Cesarean birth if a baby is breech, but a few birth centers have a provider skilled in vaginal breech delivery.

There are a number of other conditions, complications, or circumstances that vary enormously in their relative assignment of risk by different birth centers. One big variable risk factor is how many days past the estimated due date is considered acceptable before transfer to a hospital for induction of labor. Usually a full forty-two weeks of pregnancy is considered acceptable if everything else remains fine. A more questionable criterion is the estimated size of the baby (in an otherwise healthy and low-risk pregnancy). Fetal size estimates are notoriously inaccurate, and restrictions for suspected big babies vary between birth centers.

Finally, pre-pregnancy weight or weight gain during pregnancy are also considered in risking people out of birth centers, even if every index of your health is perfect. One of the NYC birth centers uses BMI as a primary tool for screening patients, asking for height and weight before scheduling a prenatal visit or answering questions about the center. Many healthy pregnant people feel unjustly excluded from birth centers by these policies.

When Susan gave birth, her birth center was inside of a hospital where she had access to the labor and delivery unit with operation rooms and high-risk doctors readily available in case she or her baby required further assistance. When the birth center is outside of a hospital, or freestanding, it usually has a transfer arrangement with a local hospital in the event that you require more medical attention or intervention than the birth center can provide. Large-scale studies of birth centers have found transfer rates to be about 10–15 percent, with less than 1 percent of transfers happening during labor for emergency reasons.[7] If you're considering a freestanding birth center, it's great to ask where they transfer to in the event of an emergency, and how long it would take for them to get you there.

Paula planned to birth in a freestanding birth center, but a diagnosis of preeclampsia resulted in an induction at a local hospital. Her midwives didn't have privileges at the hospital, although some birth center providers do, so the transfer changed both her birth location and her providers (her doula was helpful, because her support remained when everything else changed).

When Paula's midwives called with the news, she was disappointed. Giving birth in a hospital, especially being induced, was not what she'd wanted. Ultimately, she had a really positive birth experience, despite the last-minute change of venue. She transferred to a hospital with wireless monitoring so she could labor in the shower and on the toilet as she'd imagined. The induction worked more quickly than expected, and when she was bearing down with each contraction, a doctor came to check her cervix.

The doctor was surprised to find Paula fully dilated. Her amniotic sac hadn't broken and began to bulge out of her, like a small water balloon. A resident doctor who'd never seen this happen before turned to the supervising obstetrician to ask if she should break it. Hearing this, Paula reached her hands down protectively and covered the bulging sac. With the next contraction, Paula pushed her son's head out, filling the amniotic sac. It looked like a snow globe with a baby inside. The stunned resident reached her hands out just in time to catch the baby as he was born into his mother's hands. The resident supported the baby as Paula brought him to her chest. Thankfully, giving birth was the cure for her preeclampsia, as is usually the case, and Paula went home with her baby after a two-day stay in the hospital.

Many people look at birth centers as a middle ground between giving birth in a hospital and birthing at home. I'd caution against this framing. If you give birth in an in-hospital birth center, you're in a hospital with near-immediate access to everything the hospital has to offer, which is not at all like a homebirth. That said, in my experience, in-hospital birth centers have higher rates of transferring patients to the labor and delivery floor and can get bogged down in the politics and practices of the hospital. For example, NYC used to have two in-hospital birth centers, and both were routinely closed for things like staffing issues (not enough nurses) and overcrowding (birth center rooms being used for nonlaboring patients). In-hospital birth centers can easily funnel patients planning to be in the birth center to their labor and delivery floor. Knowing how often people planning to be in the birth center actually birth there can be helpful in your planning.

In a freestanding birth center, on the other hand, I've never seen issues with random closings or transferring patients to the hospital for anything other than medical reasons. That said, when you birth in a freestanding center, you're having an out-of-hospital birth, and that comes with similar risks to a homebirth. While both midwifery care and homebirth vary from state to state, a freestanding birth center may have the same resources and skills as a homebirth midwife. This means the birth center might be much less a middle ground between home and hospital, and more a homebirth not happening in your home. For some, this is a wonderful option, especially if homebirth is not legal or supported by insurance, if your home is further from a hospital, or if you'd prefer not to birth in your home. For others, it might mean you should consider the option of homebirth when weighing your decision about your birth location.

4

GIVING BIRTH
AT HOME

Many years ago I helped a family have their second baby in a planned homebirth. Her first birth was a Cesarean after weeks of her son staying in a breech position despite all attempts to move him. While this hadn't been Isabel's first choice of delivery method, she'd made peace with how he was born. Pregnant again, she planned to birth in their Brooklyn home with a local midwife.

When labor began, it was slow waves of contractions spread out over hours throughout the day. Isabel labored with her husband and son, updating the midwife and me periodically. When they were ready for me to join them, it was nearly midnight. They texted an unusual request: "When you come, can you bring firewood?" I stopped at a nearby twenty-four-hour store with bundles of firewood, and I had my cab wait while I bought some. When I arrived, Isabel was kneeling in front of her fireplace with only the light of the fire and a few small candles illuminating the room. It was a beautiful scene. Isabel seemed deep in a calm, meditative state humming through the contractions even as they grew stronger and closer together.

Later we moved upstairs into their bedroom, where her husband filled a birth tub for her to labor in. Their son was asleep in the room next door, so we whispered and tiptoed when we needed to get things or talk. Isabel moaned quietly as the contractions came. When the midwife arrived, we shared quiet embraces, and she set up her supplies. As the urge to push became more present, Isabel's husband joined her in the tub for massage and support. Their daughter was born shortly after. Within minutes, their son shuffled into the room in his pajamas with bedhead and the confusion of a child awake during the dark hours of the morning. His timing was perfect for greeting his brand-new sister as she joined their family.

Isabel's decision to birth at home is one that only about 1 percent of people in the US make. While still a very small percentage, this is nearly twice as popular as it was just over a decade ago when homebirth rates in the US were at their lowest (0.56 percent of all births).[1] Homebirth was very much the norm in this country until the last few generations when the popularity of the hospital as a birth location grew enormously. In what follows, I provide information, stories, and tools for planning a homebirth.

WHY HOMEBIRTH?

In writing this chapter, I asked a large group of people who'd chosen homebirth why they made that decision. Several people said they wanted individualized care and often referenced previous negative experiences with OBs or hospitals. One person, for example, said she'd planned to give birth in a hospital but "felt insignificant and like they had no idea who I was apart from their other patients." She didn't feel like her choices, fears, or personal history mattered. When she switched to a homebirth midwife, she immediately felt the difference: "I instantly felt respected and like I was the patient, not just the baby I was growing. I felt like I mattered and all of my fears, opinions, questions, preferences, and needs mattered."

Another person similarly told me she chose to give birth at home because she "felt safest" there and knew she would get "individualized care." Others echoed this sense of increased safety at home because of care they felt a hospital could not provide. They didn't want to be "scared" and knew they'd feel less comfortable in a hospital. One person said she feared things would "quickly get out of control" in a hospital and that "things would be thrown" at them that they would not understand. For her, negotiating consent and what that would look like in the hospital was a major concern. She felt she and her husband would be too vulnerable in that context and reflected that their midwives really made them feel safe and confident. With her midwives, "things went slow and things were comfortable at that pace."

Being in a familiar environment and being in control were also commonly cited. One woman told me, "Mainly I wanted full control in my birth in doing things the natural way and taking our time." Others listed elements of the control they were seeking, saying things like: "Allowing for me to follow my instincts and trust my body. To be in whatever position I want. To push when

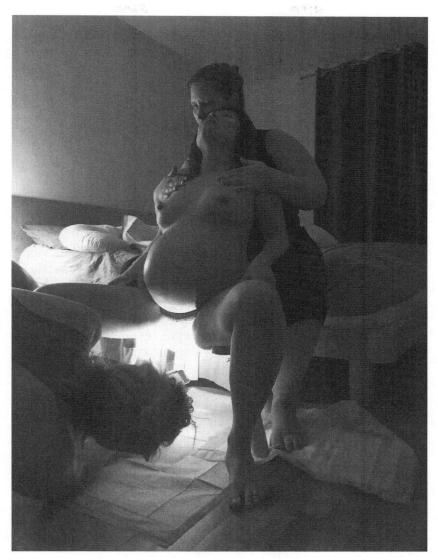

Pushing on a birth stool with midwife and doula.

I feel ready." That control was also articulated as being able to make whatever sounds they wanted, "avoiding the harsh light and sounds of hospitals," wearing their own clothing (or nothing), having whomever they wanted with them (including children), and "getting to sleep in my bed, in my apartment, with my baby and my husband that first day."

This control also extended to the treatment and care of their baby after birth. One person told me among her motivations for giving birth at home was her desire not to have her baby "taken away from me for any reason." She wanted her baby skin to skin and breastfeeding and was "scared they might say something and take her away for tests." This was a primary concern for many homebirthers—avoiding the routine policies and practices of the hospital.

For a number of my clients who've chosen homebirth for their second (or third or fourth) birth, the participation and involvement of their child/children was very important. While many families choosing homebirth don't have their children present for the birth (or like the story of Isabel's birth above, the kids sleep through it), many others do. Even for parents who don't have their older children present for the birth itself, their children often participate in the prenatal visits and become very familiar with the midwife in the months leading up to the birth. With the slower pace of prenatal visits, it's common for midwives to let kids help check the fetal heartbeat or to help inflate a blood pressure cuff.

Removing prenatal care from clinical environments means no cold stirrups at the end of the awkward bed in the exam room, and no intimidating machines or tools. Children (and their parents) are often reassured by the familiar context

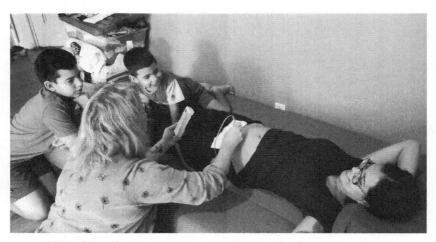

Older siblings helping during a prenatal visit with a homebirth midwife.

of the family couch or their parents' bed for prenatal visits; for many parents, this is an important step in their transition to adding another member of their family. One parent told me that she felt like the lack of sibling rivalry between her children might be related to the truly integrated experience her older son had with her pregnancy, prenatal care, and homebirth.

When I spoke with Reyna, she explained the process that led her to homebirth, stating:

> I was totally confident about birthing my baby and more comfortable being where I would not have to advocate for things like privacy, patience, and staying together. I can't remember exactly when I made the decision to hire a homebirth midwife and give birth in our apartment, but I also can't really remember a time when I hadn't already made that decision. I just knew that I wouldn't go back to the hospital to give birth.

Reyna's experience of knowing that she would birth her baby at home was very different from Sadie who had never considered a homebirth until her nursing school experiences changed her mind about where she wanted to birth. She told me:

> I'm a nurse, and the semester that I spent working as a student on the labor and delivery and postpartum floors was really eye-opening and shaped my hopes and plans for birth. Before that semester I didn't think I even wanted my husband in the delivery room with me. I was sure that if he saw an enormous baby coming out of my vagina he'd never have sex with me again. I was ambivalent as far as medications during pregnancy, C-sections and other interventions. But watching women actually going through labor without the support of their partners, actually having epidurals placed and having C-sections, having their babies removed for newborn exams and baths in the nursery really changed my views and started to give me a clearer idea of what I wanted. I realized what an extraordinarily vulnerable state labor is and how necessary it is to have an advocate and a supporter at your side. I also realized that, if possible, I wanted a less clinical birth, one where I knew everyone in the room. I wanted to feel the work of producing my baby and have that sense of accomplishment. I wanted to experience my birth, even if it involved pain, so that I knew that I had done it, not that it had been done to me.

Sadie's reasons for birthing at home were similar to many who choose a homebirth because they wanted little or no interventions. People choosing homebirth are typically enthusiastic about avoiding pain medication, IVs, and continuous fetal monitoring, and are happy to be in a nonclinical environment with people they know and trust.

The safety of homebirth is regularly debated (and the type of care provider you have matters significantly in this debate). Unfortunately, there is no high-quality data or adequate studies to really compare the safety of homebirth and hospital birth. The American College of Obstetricians and Gynecologists did recently issue a statement about planned homebirths,[2] acknowledging that in homebirth there are:

- Fewer maternal interventions such as labor augmentation with medications like Pitocin, pain medication, episiotomy, assisted vaginal deliveries (forceps and vacuums), and fewer Cesarean births
- Fewer vaginal and perineal tears, especially the most serious types (called third- and fourth-degree lacerations)
- Fewer life-threatening maternal infections

These results are partially explained by different approaches to birth among OBs and midwives and in hospitals or at home, but they're also partially a reflection of the prescreening and overall lower level of obstetric risk in people planning homebirths. When planning a homebirth, you should be carefully screened. Not all pregnancies are considered safe for homebirth; conditions such as placental problems and serious health concerns will risk you out of a homebirth. Some midwives work with people who've had a previous uterine surgery (such as a Cesarean birth) or are pregnant with twins, but many will not. Some higher-risk conditions can be identified prior to pregnancy; others, such as a breech presentation or developing preeclampsia or cholestasis, are often not identified until the end of the pregnancy after months of meeting with a midwife for prenatal care.

CARE PROVIDERS FOR HOMEBIRTH

The sense of safety, control, and slowed-down, quality, individualized care that people repeatedly cite is almost exclusively provided by midwives (although there are rare cases of homebirth doctors). There are many paths to midwifery, and licensure is widely variable. It's worth noting that midwives vary enormously in their education and training (see chapter 6). In different states this can mean a great deal about a midwife's ability to carry medications or other medical tools, their ability to work in a hospital as well as at home, and the legality of using their services (and what this might mean in the event you transfer to the hospital). Because of this, not all homebirths carry the same risks or level of safety.

When Reyna told me about the process of selecting her homebirth midwife, she recalled the counseling her midwife had offered in the interview. Her midwife told them to "remember that if anything were to go wrong, everyone would blame our choice to have a homebirth, even if it was unrelated." Reyna's midwife asked them, "Are you ready to accept that responsibility? Are you comfortable giving birth without doctors, operating rooms, and pediatricians on standby?" Understanding safety and risk, the unpredictability of birth, and the responsibility of selecting a homebirth was central to how her midwife screened clients for birthing at home.

Annie and her husband went through a similar process in their decision to birth at home and find a trusted care provider to assist them. Annie's experiences in the hospital with her dying mother convinced her she wanted to birth at home, but her husband was concerned. It was the process of researching homebirth and hiring a midwife that convinced him. Annie wrote:

> My husband . . . was way more scared to be out of the hospital. He did research in hopes of swaying me. He looked up birth centers and hospitals with midwives attending. He bought books about safe birth. He looked at the statistics. And, unfortunately for him, he found that the evidence was actually in favor of my crazy plan—hiring an experienced and loving midwife to support me at home through the entirety of my pregnancy and birth actually improves outcomes. Cesarean sections are major surgery and NYC has a really high Cesarean birth rate—staying home would help avoid this unless absolutely necessary. We struck a deal. We would find a midwife that we both completely trusted and would defer to her. If she ordered a test, we'd take it. If she wanted me on medication, I'd do it. If she said we were going to the hospital at any time, we'd go.

The sense of complete trust and building a solid relationship with a care provider that Annie spoke about was repeated throughout my conversations with people who'd planned homebirths. The quality and character of the prenatal care received from their midwives was overwhelmingly listed as among the most positive and affirming parts of giving birth at home. Gabby said:

> Each time, I would be excited waiting for the meetings with my midwife because it was so great. I loved every minute with her during my pregnancy. I cherished those prenatal appointments. They were more than a clinic visit. No waiting in a tiny waiting room or peeing in a cup. That was awful the first time. My midwife came to my home and my family, sitting with me wherever I was comfortable, asking me how I was feeling and never telling me things that stressed me out or questioning something about me. It was so lovely and I can't even describe how

meaningful this was to me. My husband totally trusted her and we talked about how amazing it was to have her.

Similarly, Ellen described her in-home prenatal care as very affirming after her previous experiences with both high-risk OBs and midwifery care in a clinic. She told me:

> She came to us for all of our appointments and this was really incredible. It was convenient, obviously, but what made it really special was how this made her a part of our family for that time. She came into our home, included my son in all of the visits by letting him help with taking my blood pressure or listening to the baby with her handheld doppler. The way she spent time with us, in our home, for every visit, gave me a level of connection to her that was so important for me.

Each of these families that I spoke with had given birth at home in New York City, where homebirth is legal; the midwives who cared for them are certified nurse-midwives who carry emergency tools like hemorrhage medications, oxygen tanks, IV equipment, and resuscitation gear. In NYC, there are hospitals nearby, and transferring to a hospital, while not totally seamless, is not particularly difficult either. In other areas of the country, however, this is not the case, and finding a homebirth midwife might be more challenging or even impossible.

About one-quarter of the time a homebirth is not attended by any medical personnel at all;[3] these are either unplanned homebirths (where they did not make it to the hospital on time) or intentionally unassisted homebirth, sometimes called "free birth." Sometimes the choice to free birth is the result of local laws that outlaw midwife-assisted homebirth, pushing people toward a birth without medical care, or because there are no homebirth midwives available in the area. In my experience, most unassisted homebirths are both planned and desired, often with a partner or family member assisting in lieu of clinical help.

Whenever I think about unassisted birth, I'm reminded of a post I read years ago on an online parenting message board where people would share everything from birth plans and tips for frugal living, to cloth diapers for sale and recipes for cake. I was pregnant with my first child at the time, and everything birth was new to me. In a forum on homebirth, a thread began about midwifery care, unassisted homebirth, and the phrase "trust birth." An anonymous poster who identified as a midwife wrote a reply I saved because it was a powerful comment on the beauty and unpredictability of birth. She'd been critiqued by a previous poster as "not trusting birth" because she advocated for having a midwife present. She responded:

I trust birth. I trust it as much as I trust any other bodily function or force of nature. I trust birth to be birth just like I trust the sea to be the sea and the wind to be wind and the rain to be rain. Which means, most of the time, I can sit back and gaze in awe at the elemental power and beauty of the sea, the rain, the wind and the birth. But I also know that within that power and beauty there is a force of nature that is beyond my, and anyone else's, control. I carry an umbrella in my car, just in case the rain demonstrates that wild, unpredictable side. I watch my kids closely when they are swimming in the sea, just in case that beautiful, blue water becomes suddenly rough or has hidden under-currents that they happily step into and suddenly pull them away. I shutter my windows and bring in my pets and remove lawn chairs when the wind threatens to become a hurricane or tropical storm. And I watch birth, ready to shelter her with my umbrella, or lift her from the currents, or really batten down the hatches and face the storm head on when that force becomes a force to be reckoned with. So, yeah, I trust birth, but even more, I respect the fact that it's a force of nature that can be wild, unpredictable, and powerful. I'm not going to say anyone who had a successful UC [unassisted childbirth] was "lucky." The odds are stacked in your favor that your birth, just like the sea or the wind or the rain, will be beautiful and safe. I don't think it's foolhardy or stupid to go swim at the beach or take a walk in a gentle summer rain, but if god forbid, you get swept away in an undertow you really don't want to be the only one on the beach who knows how to swim.

While I don't want to dismiss unassisted homebirth—I know many feel strongly about birthing without clinical care—it's not something I have experience with. As a doula I've been asked many times if I'd provide support for someone planning an unassisted homebirth, and I've thought back to this phrase—"You really don't want to be the only one on the beach who knows how to swim"—and declined. As such, all the planned homebirths I've attended were supported by midwives, or doctors if a transfer to a hospital was needed.

PLANNED VERSUS UNPLANNED HOMEBIRTH

Some unassisted homebirths are accidental: the baby arrived too quickly and was unintentionally born at home (or on the way to the hospital). This is something parents fear in the lead-up to their birth, and several couples told me they planned a homebirth because their last birth was nearly an unplanned homebirth. Babies arriving at home by mistake are most common among people who've already given birth at least once. Studies also suggest that sometimes people may be forced to stay home too long because they lack insurance or prenatal care (more than a quarter of people who had an unplanned homebirth had no prenatal care) and are planning to arrive at the hospital at the last minute in order to force the hospital to provide care.[4] As a doula, on a few occasions I've had to catch a baby who could not wait for us to get to the hospital.

One such occasion happened when Maria planned a VBAC at a local hospital but gave birth to her son minutes after I arrived at her apartment. Maria had called me months earlier when she was newly pregnant with her second baby. She very much wanted this birth to be different than her last. With her first, she hadn't known much about birth and she was unhappy with how she'd been treated. She felt unheard, hated being forced to lie still in the bed, and ultimately believed they'd moved forward with a Cesarean birth that wasn't necessary.

Maria and I had several meetings and conversations throughout pregnancy as she planned for an unmedicated vaginal birth and strategized how she'd feel about a repeat Cesarean birth if necessary. Sometimes she worried that she'd be disappointed if she was not able to birth vaginally; other times she wondered why it mattered to her so much. She'd hired a local practice known for supporting VBACs, but they used a VBAC calculator (see chapter 12 for more) that estimated a 43 percent chance she'd give birth vaginally, and they reminded her of this frequently. Her low score was the result of two factors used in the calculations: her race and her weight. We spent a lot of time talking about the problem with these calculators and my optimism that Maria would have a vaginal birth. We also talked about having a positive experience of a repeat Cesarean birth if necessary. Neither of us anticipated that I would kneel on her floor, catch her son as he slid into my hands, and wrap him with yoga pants grabbed from her nearby drawer.

A month before her due date, on Christmas Eve, she began having cramps and mild bleeding. We met at the hospital where she was seen by a midwife. They monitored her for several hours, said all was well, and sent us home to enjoy our holidays. Over the next few days Maria continued to feel crampy and uncomfortable. We talked frequently about how to cope with the discomfort and whether she should be seen by her providers again. Finally, when the pain became intolerable, she went back to the hospital. Once again, they monitored Maria for many hours and checked her cervix for signs of labor. She was now 1 cm. They sent her home after six hours of monitoring with a plan to take Benadryl, perhaps with wine, and try to sleep.

After leaving the hospital, she tried this but promptly threw up. Sleep was impossible. We talked on the phone, but having heard she was only 1 cm, she was reluctant to have me come over or return to the hospital. About three hours after she was discharged, I'd convinced her to have me come over and I took a cab to her apartment. I walked into her bedroom, greeted by her older son—up past bedtime and so excited—and found her laboring hard. I immediately said we needed to get her dressed and into the car. Labor was rapidly progressing; ideally, we'd have already been at the hospital. I pressed on her hips, coached her breathing, and quickly pulled on her pants and boots.

Dressed and ready to head to the car, she leaned onto her bed for one last contraction before facing the stairs. With this contraction her water broke, soaking the pants and shoes we'd just gotten on, and she yelled that she felt the baby coming. I pulled down her wet pants while her partner called 911. With the next contraction, her son was born into my hands, seven minutes after I walked in the door. Maria had the unmedicated VBAC she had hoped for—in a very unplanned and unpredictable way!

Maria's birth was unusual—most homebirths are planned in advance. That said, birth is unpredictable and there's always a possibility you could have an unplanned out-of-hospital birth, especially if you have a history of fast labors or you live far from where you're planning to birth.

THE LOGISTICS OF HAVING A HOMEBIRTH

If you're planning a homebirth, many of your questions are probably about the logistics of what you need, how to prepare, and what to watch out for. I've worked with clients who've worried that their home is too small to birth in (it isn't, you don't need more space to birth in than you have for living). Many people have worried their neighbors might call the police, confusing the sounds of labor for someone being murdered (they won't, labor doesn't usually sound like someone is in trouble). In my experience, most people don't even notice the sounds of labor through the walls; those who do often realize it is labor, having seen their neighbor's growing belly. One client gave her neighbors earplugs, gift cards to a wine shop, and a sweet note in preparation for her birth to help alleviate her fears that the sounds of labor (and the cries of her baby) would bother them.

Turning your space into your ideal place to labor and birth can be a fun project during the latter part of pregnancy. It can be a great project to think about what you'd like to do during labor, how you'll manage contractions, and what will make you feel calm and confident. You might want to labor on your toilet, for example, so having that space free and clear might be desirable. You may want to get a yoga ball to sit on or drape yourself over during contractions (and it can be nice prenatally as well). If you have children, the yoga ball can be a fun toy, but be careful they don't launch themselves over the ball face-first!

You might want to labor or birth in a tub. If you don't have a bathtub or it's quite small, you'll need to arrange to buy, borrow, or rent one during the month around your due date. If you get a tub, make sure you test it out to get a sense for how big it is (they are usually at least five to six feet in diameter) and where you want to put it. Ideally there is space on all sides of the tub so your birth team can reach you while you're inside. When picking a spot for the tub, remember that you'll need the tub to be reasonably close to the water source (usually a sink or shower) and the drain spot (usually a toilet) and you'll need to buy the right length hoses to reach. As well, having the tub near your bed or somewhere to lie down can be helpful in the event you give birth in the water. Shortly after you give birth, it's nice to move to a soft place to rest with your baby and best if you don't have to travel too far to get there.

Testing your tub is also important to make sure it's fully functional. Sometimes a tub has a leak or you discover you lack a necessary part to fill or drain it. I once assisted in a homebirth where the couple had not done a test run in advance, and we discovered after the birth they had no way to drain the tub. It took two very messy hours to bail out all the water with pots!

It's also good to check on your hot water supply. For Mina, after taking a hot shower to help cope with the contractions, she wanted to move to the tub but there was no more hot water. She found herself in a shallow pool of warm water with her birth team making frenzied trips between the kitchen and the tub with pots of boiling water. She recalled that the scene, while not ideal, made her laugh even with the intensity of labor.

If you have pets, you might want to make plans for their care. Having your pets around during labor can be a great source of comfort, or they can be difficult and a distraction, especially if labor or added people in your home is stressful for them. And, in the event of a transfer, you'll want to know their needs are being met.

You'll also want to have a wide variety of supplies on hand for your birth. The items you might want to have for a homebirth include:

- Most midwives will have you order a birth kit they have prepared that includes things like gloves, chux pads to absorb fluids, a bulb syringe to suction the baby, a clamp for the cord, disposable underwear and menstrual pads, a peri bottle for cleaning yourself, and a measuring tape and thermometer to assess your baby. Your midwife might also give you a list of other supplies to have on hand, so check in with them.

- At least one pair of sheets for your bed that are not special (as they may get messy). You'll want a mattress cover of some sort to protect your mattress from fluids during labor, birth, and postpartum (even if you're not planning to give birth in bed). I like to prepare the bed with a set of sheets, followed by a mattress cover, followed by another set of sheets. This makes it quick and easy to clean the bed after the baby has arrived.
- About six to eight clean towels—again, ideally not towels you're attached to, as they may get very soiled. A few washcloths can also be helpful. If you only have six to eight towels for your household, you'll want a few more since it's ideal to set aside a pile of towels for birth.
- At least two to three large black garbage bags are very useful for a homebirth. I usually set up one as the garbage, and we use that to toss out chux pads, exam gloves, emptied juice boxes, and whatnot. The second one I set up for the very soiled towels and sheets. Some people then launder these; others opt to throw them away.
- You'll need a container to put your placenta in (bowl, Tupperware, ziplock bags). Depending on your plans for the placenta, this container might vary, but no matter what your plans are, you'll need somewhere for it to go.
- When you give birth at home, it's even more important to have plenty of food and beverages on hand for you during labor and after you give birth (and also for your team). If you usually have an empty fridge, you'll probably want to change this.
- For your baby, you'll need to have clean blankets, newborn clothing, and diapers to dress and wrap them in a few hours after birth. You'll also likely want to have all of the various things people purchase in advance of their babies arriving such as a car seat, a place for the baby to sleep, baby carriers for babywearing, and more.
- Many people get a tarp or shower curtain liner for under their birth tub (or as a mattress cover). These can be helpful, but be warned, new plastic often has a strong odor at first. Consider opening it in advance and airing it out so this smell isn't present at your birth.
- You really can never have too much toilet paper at a homebirth. Whatever seems like a reasonable amount for your household, consider buying twice that.

You'll want to make sure you have a clear plan for any other children in your family. For some this means having friends, family, or a babysitter take care of a child away from home if the plan is for them to not be present. Carla recalled

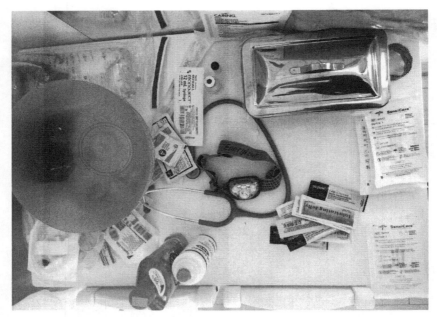

A children's table set up with supplies for a homebirth.

feeling relieved when her daughter left the house because she felt more free to labor without her daughter. In Sydney's case, she wanted her daughter there and loved letting her daughter get in the birth pool to splash and play. I strongly advise you have at least one person who's there exclusively for the sibling(s) so they have the option to leave if desired, have snacks or meals if needed, read books or play games with an adult's attention, and be cared for in the event a transfer to the hospital is needed. Your children are rarely allowed to come to the hospital (although this is a good question to ask), and having your support people stay home during a transfer might be upsetting to you.

TRANSFERRING TO A HOSPITAL

Part of homebirth preparation should be planning for the possibility of a transfer in the event that homebirth is no longer a safe option (or after the birth, if you or your baby needs more support). Sometimes this happens weeks before labor or birth, because tests have confirmed you are no longer low risk, and you have time to establish a relationship with a hospital-based midwife or doctor. Other times this happens during labor or after the baby is born, and there's little time to plan. Knowing in advance what to expect can help make a transfer more smooth and less scary.

In establishing your transfer plans, you'll want to find out what your midwife's role will be after a transfer, and who will take over your care in the new location. In my experience, some midwives will stay with you during a transfer and assist you in an advisory capacity even if they don't have clinical privileges; other midwives will discontinue care after a transfer. The care you receive from your midwife might also depend on your stage during transfer. For example, in the event you transfer to a hospital before labor has begun, your midwife is less likely to continue providing support than if the transfer takes place during labor or after you've given birth.

You may also want to pack a small bag in case you need to transfer to the hospital (see "Packing your bag" following chapter 8). And, it might be helpful to plan how you'll get to a hospital, if necessary. An ambulance is an option, but, depending on the circumstances, it can be slower. Will your midwife drive you? Someone else? Is a cab an option (depending on where you live)? And, make sure the person responsible for driving knows how to get there.

When I talked with new parents who planned a homebirth but ultimately gave birth in a hospital, one lesson several of them mentioned was coming to terms with the idea that you could really believe in homebirth and want it badly, but still not have it work. Sometimes wanting it was not enough. This is a response to the frequent emphasis in homebirth stories that's placed on emotional or psychological blocks that hold up labor progress. For example, Inez transferred postpartum when her placenta didn't come out. She said her doula told her repeatedly that she needed to "stop holding on to the placenta" and "let it go." Inez was unhappy with the assumption that it was her fault her placenta hadn't come out. Sometimes what's going on in our head has an impact on labor progress and can usefully be addressed to move forward. Other times, complications have nothing to do with psychological or emotional factors.

BIRTHING AT HOME

When Lindsay described her homebirth, she noted the contrast to her previous experience of traveling to a hospital, stating, "From my lofty position on my yoga ball I felt like a conductor and began to orchestrate the setting up of the living room between my contractions. I was telling my sister and boyfriend what to clean, what to move, where the supplies were." She continued, recalling that she smiled at one point, "thinking about how awesome it was to be doing this in my living room rather than making sure that my hospital bag was packed and getting dressed." With her first birth, she had a taxi driver who was too talkative on the way to the hospital, and in her homebirth, she was "filled with gratitude at not having to move from my apartment."

Similarly, Jean recalls her birth as a beautiful experience, highlighting the nonclinical setting and her feelings when her baby arrived. She told me:

> My bedroom leads to a backyard patio, but during the labor I was hot and kept the door closed with the air conditioner on high. After my daughter was born, my midwife was worried it was too cold in the room so we opened the back door to let in the summer heat. I remember there were birds chirping and the sunshine was streaming into the room. I was in my bed with my baby on my chest and it was the absolute best feeling imaginable. I remember her placenta sitting in a salad bowl—another reminder that birth is normal and this did not need to be a clinical experience.

Clara echoed these sentiments, telling me that "giving birth in my own home—even when it was a tiny apartment—was great. It felt so good to be in my own home, my own space, and to have time to bond and nurse uninterrupted. I am so happy that my babies were received by loving respectful people in a calm environment."

On a late spring morning, just before dawn, Noa gave birth to her second child at home. There were seven women in her bedroom—Noa, her wife, her midwife, her midwife's assistant, Noa's sister, Noa's cousin (a birth photographer), and me. A nurse at a local hospital, Noa knew exactly what a hospital or birth center would offer, and she chose homebirth. She labored on a yoga ball in the doorway to her bathroom, eventually moving to her bed. Hanging on the wall was a needlepoint that read, "Females are strong as hell." In that moment, with Noa working hard, minutes from meeting her baby, the needlepoint reminded me of Professor Laura Stavoe's quote: "There's a secret in our culture, and it's not that birth is painful. It's that women [and all birthing people] are strong."

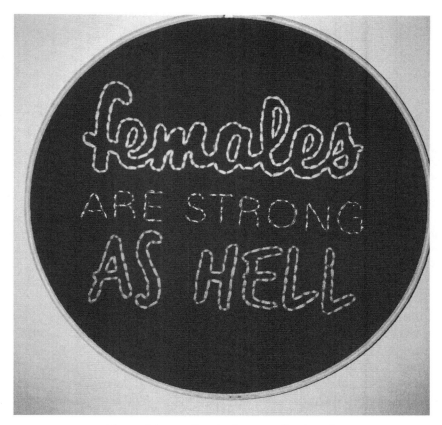

Photo of the needlepoint from my client's wall.

SELECTING A
BIRTH LOCATION

- When you imagine where you would like to give birth, what is that place like? Are there any key features of this place that you already know are important to you?
- What is available locally or within a reasonable distance? Are there multiple hospitals? Is there a birth center or multiple birth centers? Is homebirth legal, and are there any care providers in your area? You can exclude anything you already know you're not interested in and then begin researching the options that remain.
- If the options you'd like are not available locally or within a reasonable driving distance, is relocating temporarily to another area an option for you? (For example, is there a birth location near your family that you'd prefer?)
- What is the insurance coverage arrangement with this location? Does any procedure require preapproval of insurance? What will your out-of-pocket costs be?
- What types of care providers are available at this location? Obstetricians? Family practice doctors? Midwives? What credentials do the midwives have, and what do those mean? Are there residents and medical students offering care at this location?
- Do you have control over which providers you'll see at this location? Are you comfortable with everyone who will care for you? For example, if you have a preference such as only being treated by female care providers, working with a care provider of color, having a queer- or trans-supportive care provider, or working

with a body positive care provider, knowing if you can control who will be there might be important.

- What are the policies and routine procedures during birth and postpartum at this location? This might include questions about fetal monitoring, mobility, eating or drinking, required treatments for a newborn, the number of support people you can have, or separation from your baby, among others.
- What types of pain medications are available for labor or afterward? In out-of-hospital settings these might be entirely unavailable or minimally available (which might be a pro or a con depending on your preferences).
- What is the method of induction at this birth location, and how often are inductions performed? When and why might an induction be considered? For planned out-of-hospital births, how and where would an induction be done if transfer is needed? Who will care for you in that scenario?
- How often are interventions (such as breaking the water, giving Pitocin, or performing an episiotomy) performed at this birth location? What is the Cesarean birthrate?
- Does the birth location provide access to comfort measures like showers or tubs, birth balls or peanut balls, and tools for aiding in pushing such as squat bars or birthing stools? Do providers there encourage the use of these comfort measures and tools?
- Does this location have options for seeing high-risk doctors? Is there a neonatal intensive care unit (NICU) available? If they are not routinely available, how are they accessed if needed?
- What are the policies of the location regarding lactation support (if this is your plan)? For example, are there lactation consultants and classes, is there other chest/breastfeeding support, is rooming-in with the baby encouraged, is formula use with chest/breastfed babies minimized to cases of demonstrated medical need, is donor milk available?
- What types of labor and postpartum support are available? Does this location provide labor support (volunteer doulas or nurses), and if so, what roles do they play? How many support people are allowed at this location? Are there policies that restrict the number of support people, relationships of those support people, or hours when support is available for labor or postpartum? Can you have your other children with you if you'd like?

II

BUILDING YOUR BIRTH TEAM

How you're treated in birth matters enormously, perhaps even more than the specifics of what happens. This is a point I can't emphasize enough and something so critical to consider as you plan for your birth. Recently I met with a new client, Erin, only a few weeks into her second pregnancy. She was researching her options, planning for a more positive birth experience than her first. Erin wrote in her initial email about her first birth: where she had given birth, how she'd been treated, and how she felt about it. Her message to me clearly highlighted the importance of your support team and being treated well in labor. She said:

> There were so many people, and I knew they were largely there to help me (although a few were definitely there to just learn from "my case"), but there was also really no one there for us. They couldn't take the time to explain things to us. I saw different doctors every time so no one knew who I was, and most of their time was spent looking at charts.
>
> When I think back on my first birth, I really have no idea what happened or why. I still have so many questions about what was going on in the room. . . . So little was explained to me, and frankly my head wasn't in the best place to understand things, so even when they were being explained I couldn't think. I could not ask the right questions to help me actually understand what all of that meant. . . . They speak in medical terms and about things I'm not familiar with.
>
> In so many ways, my birth was a good birth, but for me, it really wasn't a good experience. I had a healthy baby, born vaginally, and I'm grateful for that but I wasn't treated well and I won't go back there. I want to do things differently this time.

Erin's words are a reminder that even when everything is good from a clinical perspective, that doesn't always translate to having a positive experience. A positive experience is more often about how you're treated and supported in birth; about being able to make decisions and understand what's happening; and about feeling in control, respected, and informed throughout the process. That is what Erin missed the first time and what she was seeking in her second birth.

One of the strongest messages from both of my own births, and the hundreds of births I've attended since, is the incredible value and importance of thoughtfully building your birth team. Surround yourself with people who you know will believe in you and support you, who will keep you safe, and who will treat you with respect. This is critical no matter what your plans are or what location you've selected.

Your birth team includes your clinical team and your nonclinical support people. Your clinical team might include doctors, midwives, residents, medical students, anesthesiologists, nurses, physician's assistants, birth assistants, and more. Part of the decision about who's on your team is made when you pick a birth location, a reason to carefully consider location, but even within those constraints, there are a lot of options for who you'll have caring for and supporting you. If you give birth in a birth center, for example, it might be staffed by midwives and birth assistants. A hospital might have residents and medical students, physician's assistants, nurses and nursing students, anesthesiologists, and other clinical staff as well as midwives or doctors, and you may only be in partial control of who is there. In a homebirth, you'll likely have the greatest control in selecting your team, although some midwives use assistants who you might not meet in advance.

When I interviewed people about their birth teams, asking who was there and why, so many people only mentioned their emotional support team—their partner, spouse, friend, mother, sister, doula. One woman told me she was only going to have her husband at her birth because it was the start of their family and she wanted an intimate experience for the two of them. Another person said she only wanted her partner because she didn't need "an audience" for her birth. I questioned them further: "Did you have a doctor or a midwife or just your husband/spouse? Was there a clinical team there?" People often laughed at this question and then told me about the various clinical providers they had initially not considered part of the list of people they'd had for their team. I understand the distinction they were making, clinical versus nonclinical. I want to keep clinical providers and medical staff in how your team is imagined because ultimately, thoughtfulness about who you want to include definitely extends to them.

Who you pick for your nonclinical team should be entirely within your control and can include people such as a spouse, partner, girlfriend or boyfriend, a friend, a coparent, family members, or a doula, among others. In my experience, most birth teams are composed of the clinical staff (however big or small that is) and one to three nonclinical support people. As a doula, I've attended births with teams that varied enormously including an acupuncturist invited to help with pain relief, a spiritual adviser, various friends or family who were doulas-in-training themselves, children, the parents adopting the child, videographers or photographers, and more. Your nonclinical team should be up to you, but in selecting it you should check on any constraints imposed by your location or clinical team. Many hospitals, for example, will allow two to three support people in a labor room and one to two people in an operating room. You should also make sure that you and your partner, if you have one, are on the same page about who else you are inviting to be at that birth. If you find someone very comforting but your partner does not get along with them at all, this can make for a less ideal birth team.

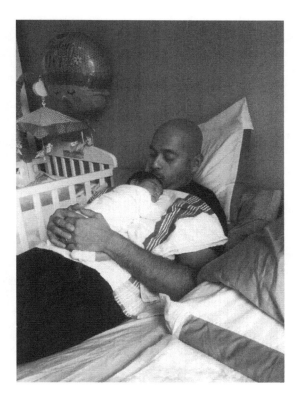

New father with his baby.

I've been to births where the team was incredible, and it felt like an amazingly supportive environment for my client. That's certainly the goal no matter who you've picked for your team. I've also been to births where I was shocked by how unsupportive and inappropriate some of the birth team were (I've been asked on occasion to help remove someone or see if a change of nurse or resident could be negotiated). In some cases people felt obligated or bullied into having people with them during birth who they didn't want present—a medical student or a mother-in-law, for example. Who you pick is a choice you should make carefully in order to surround yourself with people who help you feel calm, confident, and capable.

Many years ago I helped Katerina and Nik have their second baby in a planned VBAC, and the support Katerina's mother gave at a critical time was an excellent example of how valuable the right nonclinical team can be. Having a vaginal birth after her previous Cesarean was important to Katerina. When labor began, I joined them at home, and later in the day we traveled to the hospital. The midwives met us there and attended to her clinical needs while Nik and I continued with massage, breathing, and coaching Katerina through contractions. At some point her mother arrived at the hospital, excited by the news. Hospital policy was two support people in the room—in this case that was Nik and me—but the staff were relaxed about Katerina's mother visiting a few times.

When Katerina began pushing, it was difficult for her, as it had been the first time. The baby moved slowly. She worked hard to move the baby lower and lower over the course of the next couple of hours. Both Katerina and the baby were getting more exhausted. The baby's heart rate was dipping lower with each contraction, a sign that her baby was stressed by the process. This increased the number of medical personnel in the room and the volume as more and more people tried to urge and encourage Katerina to push harder, stronger, more. It became chaotic.

The door to the room was open, but they'd pulled a curtain across the doorway. Katerina's mother had been in the waiting room when Katerina started pushing, but as more time passed, her mom began to worry. She came to her daughter's room and heard the chaos of beeping monitors, doctors and nurses yelling instructions, and her exhausted daughter. With the curtain pulled, we did not even know she was there.

Very exhausted and frustrated, Katerina declared: "I can't do it! You need to cut this baby out of me!" Through the next contraction, she refused to push and yelled, "Cut this baby out!" repeatedly. Thankfully, that was not the most viable option at that point given how low the baby was and how much Katerina wanted a vaginal birth. After quiet conversation, Katerina agreed to keep pushing, and her midwife called in another doctor to help with a vacuum. Everyone believed this would work, but Katerina was warned if the vacuum failed, they'd convert to a Cesarean.

Overhearing her daughter breaking down and the negotiation to try a vacuum-assisted birth, her mother finally spoke through the curtain, which was a very *Wizard of Oz*-like moment. "Honey, I know you're tired, but you have to do this *now*. You have to push this baby out. I *know* you can do it." Her mom's voice really cut through all of the turmoil and confusion in the room (and in Katerina's head) and helped her become focused. She was visibly relieved to hear her mom's voice and seemed more determined with her mom's insistence she could do it.

With the vacuum in place and the OB ready to pull while she pushed, a contraction came, and she dug deep to give some of her best pushes. Within minutes Katerina and Nik's daughter was born, letting out a huge scream to announce her presence in the world. Katerina burst into tears, turned her head toward the curtain-covered door, and said, "I did it Mom!" with pride. When her mom replied, "I know! You did it!" you could hear tears in her voice. Her mom came around the curtain and saw her granddaughter for the first time. This moment remains a sweet moment of labor support, and an example of what it means to have people you trust and who believe in you.

Similarly, for Raquel, her mother's help was so valuable. She was very near to fully dilated with an overwhelming urge to bear down, but her doctor wanted her not to push yet. Her mother stepped in with breathing techniques she'd used during Raquel's birth decades earlier. Her mom helped her focus on exhaling through contractions for twenty minutes until her doctor agreed it was time to push.

In my own first birth, my mother was able to take photographs that are so special to me, and I will never forget the homemade sandwich she fed me after I gave birth. Other people I interviewed also spoke in praise of having their mothers, mothers-in-law, aunts, sisters, and friends as part of their birth team. One woman told me that her partner passes out from blood, so her mom was with her through her Cesarean birth. Another new mom called her mother an expert—she'd birthed six kids of her own—and said she was happy to have her mom as a labor coach for her all of her births.

Increasing numbers of pregnant people also turn to doulas as advocates and labor coaches.[1] Rose was five weeks pregnant when an ultrasound resulted in the surprising news that her uterus was bicornate—shaped differently with two "horns" in a more heart-shaped appearance than normal, leaving less room for the baby and resulting in a higher risk of premature and Cesarean birth due to breech positioning. She said, "With so many things already feeling out of our control, I wanted to have the healthiest pregnancy possible, to control everything I could control." She hired a doula to help support them on the "unpredictable road ahead." Rose said her pregnancy was "a test" for her with "so much powerlessness and lack of control, a weird sense of uncertainty, and the fear of our daughter coming early." Having a doula was "an incredible asset" and a big part of why she felt good about her birth and at peace with everything that needed to happen.

For Pamela, the decision to not have a doula was "very straightforward." She felt super connected to her doctor, a solo practitioner who promised he would guide them through the experience from the moment they arrived at the hospital until after her baby was born. Her tour of the hospital was a great opportunity for her to meet several of the nurses in labor and delivery, and she felt very at ease with how "kind and welcoming" they all seemed. The extra expense and extra personality of adding a doula to the team felt "unnecessary and undesirable." She and her husband read several birth books, took a weekend class to make sure they knew all the basics, and described their experience of birth as really intimate, supported, and peaceful. Pamela built a birth team she felt comfortable with, and it helped her have a positive experience.

Inviting someone to your birth who's helpful and supportive definitely can make for a more positive experience. The opposite can also be true: inviting people who aren't helpful or supportive can create unwanted drama or conflict during birth. Being really clear with family, friends, or your doula about what you expect their role to be is helpful. It's also good to warn people that you might change your mind in labor.

Similarly, understanding who might be in the room or involved in your care at your birth location is valuable. Medical students, for example, are often in hospitals as part of their training, but you can request no medical students be involved in your care if you prefer. Some clients have had strong preferences for only having women on their clinical team, and in hospitals in particular, this can require some negotiation. In homebirth or at a birth center, your midwife might have a midwifery student and should talk with you about whether you're comfortable with the student being present or not. In a hospital or birth center there might also be student nurses eager to observe your birth and assist. For some, offering students a chance to learn during their birth feels like a wonderful gift, and for others it feels like an invasion of privacy in an intimate moment. Both are valid feelings, and talking about who you'd like present can be helpful.

Being thoughtful about who you invite to your birth can be overwhelming and confusing when you don't know very much about the differences between the various care providers and support people you can choose to have assist you. In the next three chapters—on doctors, midwives, and doulas, respectively—I'll help you navigate the differences between types of care providers, things you might want to consider in selecting your doctor or midwife, the additional support people or clinical staff who might accompany your care provider, how the support of a doula might be helpful, and other questions to consider as you build your birth team. In what follows I address questions such as:

What is the difference between a doctor and a midwife?
What is the difference between a midwife and a doula?
Are all midwives trained and licensed the same way?
Does this change how they practice or what is available to me with a midwife?
What can a homebirth midwife do in emergencies?
How does this compare to being with a midwife or doctor in the hospital or in a birth center?
Does picking one care provider afford me access to anything specific I might find desirable?
Conversely, does it limit my access to any options, treatments, or technologies?
What other clinical support people might be at my birth, and what should I expect from them?
Why are doulas important if I already have a doctor or midwife?
Are doulas differently trained, and what does it mean if they are certified or not?
What obstacles (legal, financial, availability, etc.) might I encounter in seeking care?

Throughout each chapter there's information and stories aimed at helping you select a team you feel safe and supported by. Returning to the three Cs of childbirth—control, choice, and consent—can help you as you navigate picking your team. Finding your people, whoever they are, is about honoring who *you* are, what *you* want in your birth experience, and how *you* feel.

5

WORKING WITH A DOCTOR

Leah's first two pregnancies ended in complicated miscarriages. Those experiences informed her decision-making in future pregnancies. She'd started with a gynecologist that she loved but, after becoming pregnant, found out her doctor no longer practiced obstetrics and couldn't help her. Leah then followed the advice of a friend who loved their doctor, but her experience with that doctor was terrible. She tried another doctor but was upset when they treated her coldly during a miscarriage. She said, "These experiences had me bouncing from doctor to doctor, many of whom surprised and hurt me with misdiagnoses, brusque treatment, an unwillingness to listen, and a sometimes paternal patronizing that dismissed my medical concerns and physical discomfort as nothing more than 'sad pains.'"

Frustrated and overwhelmed, Leah reached out to her gynecologist for a recommendation. He sent her to a high-risk doctor he thought might be a match, but that doctor was not able to perform the procedure she needed. He sent her to "a younger doctor in the practice who became my OB and will be for the rest of my life. She was amazing and the practice was amazing." Her new doctor was patient, took her time during appointments, and "listened when I explained what was going on and when I asked questions." In their conversations, her doctor explained things clearly, referred to recent research, and always "understood and explained the risks and benefits of different procedures or interventions." Plus, "she was available always. I mean always. I could text her questions or concerns, and she'd get back to me quickly. If she was away, her secretary would put me in touch with someone else who could help."

For Leah, now pregnant again and scared, it was so important to have someone who listened, gave her all the information to make choices with, and was available. She described her pregnancy as really challenging: the relief that there was finally a "heartbeat on the monitor at every visit" and the doubt she couldn't shake even at twenty-eight weeks or thirty-six weeks. Working with her doctor provided comfort and helped her manage the emotional and physical turmoil.

Leah also felt confident about the other doctors in the practice who shared on-call time with her doctor. For both the birth of her son and, two years later, her daughter, her doctor was not on call. Instead, a colleague was there to assist when Leah went into labor. Leah said they were all "professional, personable, and relaxed." Since they were high-risk doctors, she felt they had "seen it all" and "little challenges did not freak them out."

When Leah's first baby needed to be born via a Cesarean birth, she felt confident this was not just "an easy, quick solution" for them but a necessary intervention. Hours of labor had been punctuated with scary decelerations in her baby's heart rate. She recalled the final deceleration, "one that required a full flip over onto my hands and knees and medicine to stop my contractions." That last one solidified her feelings: "I wanted my baby to be healthy; I didn't want to hear his heart go down to a slow whisper again; I wanted him out and cared for; I wanted him to be okay." A few minutes later in the operating room, he was out, and while he needed a few days of help in the NICU, he was healthy and safe.

Almost two years later (and a month before her due date), when Leah's water broke in the middle of "a VERY fancy dinner" for her husband's law firm, she lined the backseat of a cab with linen tablecloths from the restaurant and went to the hospital. Again, she felt so confident about her care. She said, "All of the rules many doctors make for women trying to have vaginal births after Cesarean births—about monitoring, epidurals, Pitocin—were guidelines for them, not dogma." She had two very different births with "every intervention we learned about in our birth class," but she still loved both of her birth experiences.

Leah is similar to the vast majority of pregnant people in the US in that she hired a doctor and gave birth in the hospital her doctor (and colleagues) had privileges at. Nearly four million people give birth every year in the US, and about 85 percent are attended by a doctor:[1] an obstetrician usually, but also perinatologists (or maternal fetal medicine doctors, a specialized branch of obstetrics), and occasionally family practice doctors. Many people see doctors for their prenatal care without realizing any other type of provider, such as a midwife, is even an option.

As Leah's story highlights, doctors, like all of us, have a wide range of personalities and approaches, so finding someone who's a match for you is important. It took Leah several doctors before she found a great match. If you're wondering if working with a doctor is right for you or trying to find the right doctor to support you, this section will help.

WHAT TYPES OF DOCTORS ATTEND BIRTHS?

When I interviewed new parents about the process they went through in finding a doctor to support them, it wasn't uncommon to hear they'd been surprised and disappointed to find that the doctor they'd been seeing prior to the pregnancy couldn't support them. Theresa, for example, recalled that before she got pregnant, she had a gynecologist she'd seen for years and really loved. When her doctor stopped taking her insurance, she stayed, paying out of pocket. She told me, "I was really excited to have a baby with her!" Unfortunately, when Theresa got pregnant, she was devastated to find her doctor didn't attend births. Theresa said, "I had imagined she would be the one with me through my birth, but that was no longer possible."

Your gynecologist might offer a full range of reproductive health care outside pregnancy but transfer your care to another doctor or a midwife for pregnancy and birth. If you're planning to get pregnant and like your current provider, double-check that they're able to care for you in pregnancy. Also check that they attend births (some doctors will see you in pregnancy but have colleagues attend your birth). If they're not able to care for you or attend your birth, you might start your search for a new provider immediately. No need to wait until you're pregnant!

There are three types of doctors you might see for prenatal care and birth: obstetricians, perinatologists, or family physicians. Obstetrics is the field of medical study concerned with pregnancy, childbirth, and the postpartum period. Obstetricians (OBs) are physicians who assist in childbirth; but unlike midwives, who are also experts in birth, OBs are trained as surgeons.

Most people can see an obstetrician for care during pregnancy. OBs care for patients having normal, uncomplicated pregnancies and also often care for higher-risk patients. In addition to being the best care provider for a scheduled Cesarean birth, obstetricians are needed for operative vaginal deliveries (midwives don't use vacuums or forceps) and are routinely called to help with complicated vaginal repairs if more extensive suturing is required after birth.

Charlotte, for example, began her low-risk pregnancy in the care of midwives but was incredibly itchy by the end of her pregnancy. Blood tests confirmed she'd developed a liver condition called intrahepatic cholestasis of pregnancy

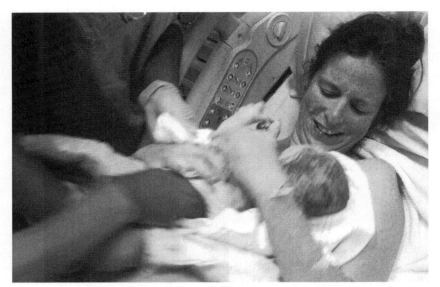

An OB handing a newborn to his mother in the moment of birth.

(ICP), and she needed to be induced. Her midwives remained her care providers, but an obstetrician was brought in to help supervise the induction. When a Cesarean birth became necessary, that OB performed the surgery. When Charlotte was pregnant with her second child, she decided to remain in the care of the obstetrician who performed her previous Cesarean rather than the midwives she had originally seen. Given her increased risk of developing ICP again and her previous Cesarean birth, she felt more confident about seeing an obstetrician for her care.

For even higher-risk clients, a perinatologist, also called a maternal fetal medicine doctor (or MFM), might be necessary. MFMs are physicians trained in the field of obstetrics but who've pursued further education in the maternal fetal medicine subspecialty. Many perinatologists work with obstetricians, comanaging the care of pregnant people who are having more complicated or risky pregnancies. If your pregnancy has been identified as high risk, you might be asked to see a maternal fetal medicine doctor in addition to your obstetrician (or you might be exclusively in the care of a maternal fetal medicine doctor, if insurance will cover it or you pay out of pocket). You might be referred to an MFM for reasons like:

- High-risk complications in a previous pregnancy
- A history of recurrent pregnancy loss

- Signs of preterm birth
- Blood pressure problems, placental problems, and problems with your heart, kidney, or lungs prior to (or during) pregnancy
- Autoimmune diseases, cancer or being a cancer survivor, infectious diseases
- Blood clotting or bleeding risk or diseases
- Seizure disorders or other brain disorders
- Certain psychiatric disorders
- Medications you might be taking that pose higher risks for the fetus/baby
- Needing surgical care while pregnant
- Being pregnant with multiples (twins, triplets, more)
- A wide variety of prenatal fetal diagnoses or complications
- Pregnant people who need fetal testing or treatment
- Postpartum complications such as infection, excessive bleeding, or seizures

Sofia's story nicely highlights a situation where an MFM might be needed (and desired). When Sofia first got pregnant, she hired midwives associated with a local birth center and planned for a low-risk, low-intervention birth. She'd been through years of trying to get pregnant on their own, testing that provided no insights into why it wasn't working, Eastern medicine and acupuncture in hopes of shifting something, IUIs (intrauterine insemination, placing sperm into the uterus during ovulation), and finally IVF (in vitro fertilization, where her egg and her husband's sperm were combined in a laboratory and the resulting embryo was transferred to her uterus). The first round of IVF worked, but unfortunately, her placenta detached from her uterus early in the pregnancy, causing lots of bleeding and the loss of that pregnancy.

Following this, Sofia said, "We got a donor egg and made an embryo from that for another round of IVF. It was an incredibly long, emotional, and expensive process but we finally got pregnant, and with twins, from that donor egg IVF." It took nine years to get to this point, but this was incredible news; she described it as "hitting the jackpot" and said the "pregnancy was really good." That said, she was nervous, and this impacted her decisions. Sofia told me:

> This past experience and the increased risks of having twins made me very anxious in my pregnancy. I was more conservative about my birth plans. With the first pregnancy, I selected midwives at a birth center, but with the twins I picked a high risk hospital with a reputation for delivering multiples vaginally. I wanted

more careful monitoring the second time around. I had a lot of ultrasounds—every two weeks—and I know there is some controversy about this but I loved having all of these extra chances to see that they were doing well. And my babies are perfect, so I feel really good about that.

I originally picked a very high risk obstetric practice (MFMs) that included a number of doctors who really like delivering twins and triplets vaginally and pride themselves in their high rate of vaginal deliveries of multiples. I wanted to have these babies vaginally, and they felt like the perfect match. Unfortunately, my insurance refused to cover their care. I was not high risk enough. At 16 weeks pregnant, I moved to a lower risk OB practice across the hall. I continued to have a high risk doctor review my case throughout the pregnancy while seeing the new OBs.

In a wonderfully ironic wrinkle, one of the high risk doctors I had wanted to work with during the pregnancy was in the hospital the day I was induced. He loves delivering multiples vaginally and always tries to be part of multiples deliveries so he joined my doctor (which was good because he ultimately ended up delivering my babies when my OB was less confident about how to manage a twins birth).

For Sofia, the increased risk from IVF, her age, the history of pregnancy loss, and a twins pregnancy made seeing a perinatologist important for her pregnancy. Unfortunately, her hope to see perinatologists for the entire pregnancy was shut down by her insurance company's refusal to cover care. Thankfully, the comanagement of her pregnancy with her obstetrician and the MFM practice she'd originally selected made it possible for her to have one of those MFMs present for her birth, supporting her in the vaginal birth of her twins.

In addition to obstetricians and perinatologists, family physicians also provide prenatal care and assist in birth, typically for low-risk pregnant people. Family physicians care for all ages of patients (the whole family) and offer preventative care (such as annual physicals, well child visits, and immunizations) in addition to treating acute and chronic health issues. A recent review suggests that less than 10 percent of family care physicians in the US currently offer obstetrical care,[2] which is bad news for families in rural areas. In areas where there are a small number of babies born, there may not be enough patients to sustain an obstetrician's practice. In these areas, a family physician is especially valuable.

CONSIDERATIONS WHEN SELECTING YOUR DOCTOR

When I asked people to talk about what they liked most about their doctor, they responded with a wide variety of traits they appreciated. For almost everyone, their doctor's training and experience was a huge source of comfort. They respected how knowledgeable their doctor was, wanted to work with someone who was evidence based (meaning they were up to date on the most recent data and practices), and trusted their skills and recommendations. Feeling listened to and included in the process was also important. People wanted their doctor to engage with them as an individual, respect their decisions, and approach them with compassion.

Telling me about one of the things she appreciated most about her doctor, Amaya recalled this story: "When he did the vaginal ultrasound at our first visit and we heard the baby's heartbeat, his face softened and he said, 'This never gets old.'"

Finding a care provider with an approach that matches your desires is important. If you're hoping to minimize tests, avoid an induction, and labor with as few of the routine procedures in the hospital as possible, then finding a provider who usually approaches pregnancy and birth this way will be important. Many people described their doctor as "noninterventionist" to summarize this approach and said they took comfort knowing their doctor would only recommend something like a Cesarean birth if it were necessary.

That said, if you appreciate having more tests and take comfort in extra precautions, that same doctor might be a terrible match for you. Andrea, for example, said that she initially liked that her doctor was "chill" but then found her doctor might have been "too chill" for her comfort level when things became more complicated. In a future pregnancy she'd want to work with someone who approached her care differently.

Martina, a midwife herself, said her search for a provider wasn't what she would have expected. She was "working a ton" in a local hospital during pregnancy, and while she and her husband talked about a homebirth, they were concerned about the financial burden. She told me:

> The year before had not been the best year for my husband's work and that meant a home birth would have been a real stretch. My aunt suggested I really consider not using all our money for the birth when I might want it to help me stay home for longer afterwards. She worried I might regret putting myself in a position where I absolutely had to go back to work right away. Ultimately, I listened to her, which I am thankful for because I was so grateful for the flexibility to stay home with my son for longer.
>
> Having decided to give birth in the hospital where I work, with a provider fully covered by my insurance, I then went about picking my doctor in a very different way than I imagine many people do. I knew all the options really well—knew their

personalities, how they work, and their skills. I'd seen them all in action and knew what to expect from each of them.

For me, my primary question then became who could I trust to operate on me in case I needed a Cesarean. That's funny I think. I am a midwife, and my one criteria was who would I be okay with as a surgeon! That was my perspective because I felt like I knew how to avoid much of the silliness—unnecessary interventions or unneeded procedures. I understand birth and I was confident about that. Given this, what I really needed was someone who I would not be freaked out to have operate on me. So, I picked a group of doctors I trusted and I had a friend who is a midwife support me during the labor.

For Martina, this was the right balance. She had a vaginal birth with an epidural, a friend and her husband for support, and a doctor from her practice managing the complications that arose during labor. Her baby showed signs of distress during labor, and afterward her colleagues told her she was "lucky" she gave birth vaginally. She said:

What I remember, though, was not that I felt lucky to have had a vaginal birth, but that I felt so lucky that my baby was ok and that everyone had been so nice to me. I felt well cared for and I trusted everyone to help me and keep me safe. I felt grateful for having that feeling the entire time, even when things were more complicated. I knew I was in good hands with my doctor and that things would be ok whatever needed to happen.

Martina went on to say that the experience of giving birth changed how she approaches her care for others as a midwife. She told me:

Every interaction that I had with the nurses and my doctor was more than respectful, it was kind. That meant everything to me. When you feel so vulnerable it's the one thing you really need to have a good experience. Kindness. Even though my birth was different than planned, I think that things could have gone exactly as I had wanted, but if it had been in hostile conditions, it would not have felt like a positive experience.

As a midwife I bring this experience with me so much now. Giving birth gave me insights that have impacted my practice. I remember how loud everything was in my own birth and as a midwife, I am even quieter than I used to be.

I remember that it was my feelings that ended up really mattering to me and not what happened. My feelings were looked after and that was so important to me. It can be hard, impossible even, to guarantee all the other things—that your birth will go as planned or that you will have the experience that you imagined wanting—but there is no reason why everyone should not feel loved and cared for regardless of what is happening in their birth. Everyone should have that experience, and I am so grateful that I did.

As Martina's story highlights, working with a birth team you trust and feel cared for by is key to having a positive experience. Her doctors provided her with the clinical care she needed but also the kindness that made her birth a really positive experience.

As you build your team, it can be helpful to find out what tests a doctor recommends or routinely performs prenatally, how often you should expect to have ultrasounds, how frequently you'll see them, how you can contact them, and what to expect for labor and birth in terms of induction policies, requirements in labor (like IVs, fetal monitoring), and how often their patients need a Cesarean birth. It can be helpful to think about how you feel about their communication style, how they touch you or treat you, and how you feel when you're with them. If you like your doctor's policy on induction and attitude toward labor, but you feel talked down to or shamed by them or their touch feels rough, for example, you might need to keep looking.

Additionally, it's important to note that many doctors work in group practices that might range in size from just two doctors or more than a dozen doctors, and you may not be able to meet the other doctors in advance. For some people, knowing the doctor who'll be with you during your birth is important; for others, it is not significant. For Theresa, she said she trusted her doctors but also was not very concerned about which one was on call when she gave birth because "the doctor was mostly not with us. He would leave the room to see other patients or talk with the other staff or add notes to my chart. I am not entirely sure what he was up to but, he was mostly not with us." She had a doula and her husband for support, and not having her provider around was fine.

Phoebe, on the other hand, began her pregnancy with an IVF doctor, and when it was time to switch to an OB, she didn't give it much thought and didn't think it mattered. She said, "My friends who liked their doctors all told me that their doctors were not even present when they gave birth because someone else was on call that day." That said, a few months into the pregnancy when she started considering her birth options, she wished she "would have put more thought into picking our doctor." She said:

The doctor we picked was too clinical and forceful and really didn't share my views, which became increasingly clear. She didn't think there were too many C-sections, for example, and made it seem like every C-section was always necessary. I knew on a gut level when I talked with her that I felt like I was losing control. I would not be making any decisions with her; I would be doing what she told me. Thankfully, our doctor announced mid-pregnancy that she was moving out of state. My wife and I considered staying with her practice and seeing the other doctors but we were ready to find someone new.

Our doula recommended a new doctor—a quirky, sweet guy with a Mr. Rogers vibe. He wasn't trying to shove any statistical meow-meow down our throats like the other doctors. He was soft-spoken, gentle, relaxed, and a solo practitioner, so I knew he'd be there.

Before we realized we would need IVF, we'd hired a midwife who advertised her work with queer families. I thought I would want a woman. I thought I would care that she totally understood our family. In the end, I did not like her or how I felt with her, but this man was very personable and kind to me. He encouraged laboring at home and supported my plan to have little intervention. He was there with us the whole time in the hospital and helped me have the birth experience I wanted.

For Phoebe, finding a solo practice doctor who would be with her during her labor ended up being more important than things she'd previously thought would matter. Although she ultimately didn't find that working with a female doctor or a queer-identified provider was important to her, her story does highlight that this might be important to you. When I met with Sam, for example, she told me that she'd never worked with a man for her reproductive health care and couldn't imagine having a male OB. In her search for a care provider, this took out all of the practices that included male providers and significantly narrowed her options.

For other clients, the gender of their care provider was not as important as other factors such as the importance of working with a doctor of color, for example, or someone with the same religious or cultural background or who speaks the same language as you. After reading about the huge disparities in safety and outcomes for pregnant people of color, Tioma told me that she hired an OB who was also black because she felt she would receive better care and be less at risk if her provider shared in her experiences of being a woman of color in the US. When Nieves was pregnant with her first baby, she felt confident about her proficiency in English while not under stress but suspected that she and her partner might prefer the option to communicate with their doctor in Spanish, their first language, during labor or if more complicated decisions needed to be made.

For Tess, who was born without arms, finding a doctor who had already supported other clients with similar bodies was really important to her. She could not imagine having to educate her provider on supporting her and instead looked to online support groups for people with bodies like hers to see which doctors others recommended. This experience was common among the fat parents I spoke with—they'd often searched online forums to find local providers who had respectfully cared for other people with bodies like theirs before meeting with anyone for prenatal care.

When Aidan began his search for prenatal care, he was particularly concerned with finding a provider who'd already worked with trans clients and wouldn't need to be educated in order to support him. He'd been encouraged by friends to seek out a midwife, but the only two midwifery practices in the area did not take his insurance. This made the option of midwifery care prohibitively expensive. He couldn't find recommendations for local doctors who had experience working with pregnant men, so he began calling the offices covered by his insurance and explaining to the person who picked up, "I am pregnant and trans. Will your office be able to respectfully care for a pregnant man?" He had a few conversations he described as "both totally awkward and really clarifying—it was clear that these offices who stumbled all over themselves trying to make sense of me and my request were not the right place for me."

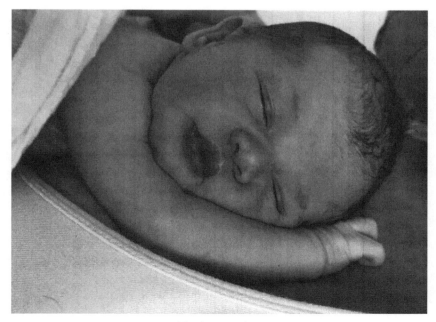

Newborn resting.

Thankfully for Aidan, after a few of these awkward phone calls, he asked his question again and was met with a simple, "Congratulations on your pregnancy. We'd love to have you as a patient. Do you know how far along you are? Would you like to schedule your first visit?" He ultimately found a practice with three doctors who were all respectful in their care and proactive about making his experience of pregnancy and birth really positive.

Whatever you're looking for in your provider and whatever your needs are in pregnancy, actively seeking out someone who's a good match from the beginning of the process will benefit you enormously. If you find yourself with a provider who feels like a bad match, it's OK to find someone else and switch to their care. Selecting the right type of doctor, with a personality and practice that matches your preferences, will help you have a positive birth experience.

INTERVIEWING A DOCTOR

If you're planning to give birth with a doctor, you might ask for recommendations from other doctors, friends, family, online forums, your doula, or others. When you're researching and meeting with potential doctors, you might ask some of these questions, whichever address things that are important to you as you make decisions about where to give birth and with whom.

TRAINING AND EXPERIENCE

- What is your training/education/experience?
- How long have you been practicing?
- Do you offer any additional services personally or through your office that might be useful for me in pregnancy or postpartum?

HOSPITAL AFFILIATIONS

- What hospital are you affiliated with?
- If there are multiple, how much choice will I have in where I give birth?

COMMUNICATION

- Are you available twenty-four hours a day, seven days a week during my pregnancy?
- If not, when are you available and not available?
- How can I communicate with you?

YOUR PRACTICE

- How many doctors are in your practice?
- Are there any midwives in your practice?
- Will I rotate between everyone in the practice for care or primarily see you?
- Will I have any choice over which provider is with me for the birth?
- Do you have residents or medical students assist with my care during labor and birth?
- What tasks do they assist with?
- What differences are there between the providers in your practice?
- What happens when you disagree with each other on the best approach?

SCREENING AND RISK

- What types of prenatal tests do you require? Recommend?
- How will you communicate the results of these tests with me?
- Are there circumstances that would require me to consult with another doctor during pregnancy?
- Are there circumstances that would require me to consult with another doctor during labor?
- Are there circumstances that would require my care to be transferred to another doctor?
- In the event of a transfer, are there doctors you recommend?

INDUCTION (ALSO SEE CHAPTER 11)

- Beyond emergent signs that an induction is necessary, at what point would you recommend scheduling an induction?
- How common are inductions in your practice? What percent of your clients do you induce?
- What induction techniques do you routinely use?
- What induction medications are available at the hospital where you practice?

CESAREAN BIRTH (ALSO SEE CHAPTER 14)

- How common are Cesarean births in your practice?
- Do you offer gentle or family-centered Cesarean birth options?
- Do you have medical students assist you during Cesarean births? What tasks do they assist with?

LABOR SUPPORT AND CHILDBIRTH EDUCATION

- Do you work with doulas? Can you recommend some?
- Do you work with birth photographers?
- Do you recommend a childbirth class to prepare? Can you recommend one?

POSTPARTUM SUPPORT

- What kind of postpartum care do you offer?
- Do you have experience with supporting chest/breastfeeding?
- Do you have a resource list for clients if I need referrals to physical therapists, lactation consultants, therapists, support groups, and so forth?

PERSONALITY/PHILOSOPHY

- Why did you become a doctor?
- What is your philosophy of birth?

BUSINESS

- Do you take insurance? What type of coverage should I expect?
- What has your previous experience been with insurance coverage?
- Does every provider in your practice also take my insurance?
- Is the hospital you are affiliated with covered by my insurance?
- How much do you charge, and by what date would the full amount be due?
- Do you accept payment plans? What is your refund policy if we switch providers?

6

WORKING WITH
A MIDWIFE

"Wait, I can have an epidural with a midwife?" Ryuko asked with confusion. We'd met because she wanted to talk through plans for her upcoming birth. She started the conversation recalling her best friend's recent birth—a water birth in a Manhattan apartment with a midwife, her husband, a doula, Ryuko, and their golden retriever. This was the only birth Ryuko had ever seen, and the experience was incredible, but she knew it wasn't how she'd give birth. For her birth, Ryuko wanted to have an epidural in a hospital. She imagined this required hiring an OB.

After telling me her preferences, Ryuko asked if I could recommend local obstetricians, believing this was her only option. I offered a list of my favorite OBs but also let her know that wanting an epidural in a hospital didn't mean she had to work with an OB necessarily.

All across the country midwives work in hospitals, expertly supporting hundreds of thousands of people giving birth, with and without epidurals. It's not uncommon for people to have inaccurate ideas about midwives—who they are, what they do, who their clients are, where they work. Often discussions about midwives involve jokes about boiling water or crystals and herbs. Partially this confusion stems from how uncommon the use of midwives has been in most of our lifetimes. I was born in the late 1970s when nearly all babies in the US were born in a hospital with a doctor. While that has changed significantly, about 85 percent of births in the US are still attended by doctors. The US is the exception in this because midwifery care is the norm in much of the world.[1]

The confusion in the US about midwives also partially stems from the wide range of types of midwives and what their varied trainings and credentials mean about where and how they practice. Midwives attended nearly all births in this country at one time—British-trained colonial midwives, enslaved West African midwives, and indigenous midwives. Midwifery wasn't a regulated practice with formal education and credentialing, but a set of skills learned from assisting a mentor. This lack of regulation continued until the 1920s when midwives found themselves being outlawed by new regulations all over the country. These laws were passed at the state level, though, resulting in the mess we have today: a patchwork of different laws, training, licensing, and oversight that are incredibly challenging to navigate as a pregnant person looking for care and weighing your options.

In what follows, I want to clarify the types of midwives, where and how they practice, and when and why you might want to hire a midwife. I begin by detailing the shared definition of midwifery care created by multiple midwifery groups in the mid-nineties: the midwives model of care. Then I discuss the history of midwifery and the various types of midwives who practice in the US (and what their credentials might mean for your birth). I turn to safety and outcomes with midwives and why you might choose midwifery care for your own birth. I also present a number of situations where midwifery care is not a good option. Throughout, I aim to dispel myths about both midwives and the people who seek their care.

THE MIDWIVES MODEL OF CARE

Recognizing that many people are confused about what modern midwifery care looks like, in 1996, several key midwifery organizations drafted a joint definition of midwifery care to share with health care decision makers and patients.[2] The Midwives Alliance of North America (MANA) identifies different "skills, tools, language, underlying beliefs, interventions, and power relationships"[3] as key areas where midwives, and their model of care, can differ from other providers and models of care. Midwifery care is "uniquely nurturing," centering the belief that pregnancy and birth are normal life events, not medical crises. For low-risk patients, midwives can provide all the prenatal care and birth support a doctor can provide with a model of care that includes physical well-being, as well as psychological and social well-being.

Natasha described this attention to her physical, psychological, and social well-being in her prenatal visits, saying that the focus was on "more than the baby" with conversations that were personal and relaxed. Natasha said, "I've been asked about my sleep, my emotions, how I am eating, and changes to my body." Tina described her connection with her midwives as professional but also "caring and intuitive," highlighting the experience of whole-person care.

Similarly, when Molly told me about her births, she spoke about her initial experiences with a high-risk doctor and her subsequent move to midwifery care. For Molly, the difference in care was "night and day." She said birth was one of the most profound and powerful experiences of her life and she wanted "a provider who was compassionate about that." She didn't want five-minute meetings, statistics on risks, or tests ordered without conversation—her experience with her doctor—but instead wanted "a care provider who was part of that journey with me."

Beyond this commitment to holistic care, another core principle of the midwives model of care is minimizing technological interventions. This doesn't mean interventions such as IVs, medication, epidurals, or inductions are not available with midwives but rather that midwives use these interventions as little as possible. If staying hydrated by drinking fluids during labor is possible, for example, midwives tend to opt for that over IV fluids. If a hot shower can provide pain relief, most midwives will work to make that available. If there is no health concern, midwives tend not to schedule inductions, suggesting nonmedical ways to get labor started.

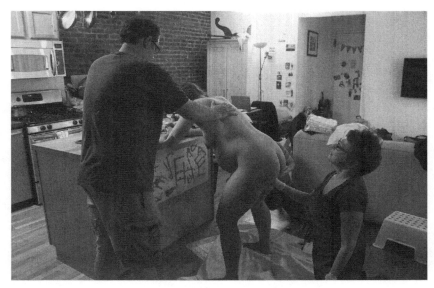

Midwife assisting with pushing at a homebirth.

73

In the hundreds of births I've attended, I've found this to be true: compared to doctors, midwives generally schedule fewer inductions, midwives give fewer medications to speed up labor, and midwives are slower to suggest a Cesarean birth when labor or pushing has been long. As well, midwives are more likely to suggest pushing in a variety of positions, more likely to use nonmedical techniques to increase the frequency or strength of contractions (movement, position change, or nipple stimulation), and are more likely to advocate for clients to stay with their support people and newborn.

Providing individualized care, education, counseling, and support is another core principle of the midwives model of care. This commitment is part of what MANA references when it says midwives maintain a different power relationship with clients. Carrie told me she worked with midwives because they helped her understand her options and respected her choices. Similarly, Natasha said that working with midwives allowed her to be "the driver" of her care, with her midwife empowering her to "accept and decline anything." Kaitlin said the best thing about her midwifery care was that it was all truly in her own hands. Bell said her midwife didn't "overdo it on the panic" and gave her "more choices" throughout her pregnancy and birth. Marissa told me her midwives hadn't been strictly focused on numbers (dates, weights, percentiles, tests) but instead had focused on her whole person, which made her feel both safe and cared for. This individualized care, counseling, and support is central to the model of care.

A final core piece of the midwives model of care is providing appropriate referrals to obstetricians when needed. Midwives provide prenatal, postpartum, and well care for healthy, low-risk patients. If a patient stops being healthy, or a pregnancy becomes high risk, transferring to an appropriate doctor is how midwives care for patients. For example, when Terry's twenty-week ultrasound revealed a rare fetal heart condition, the midwives at the birth center she'd planned to give birth at explained that this was no longer an option. They referred Terry to a high-risk obstetrician. While Terry was disappointed, the need for an OB in a high-risk hospital was clear, and she was able to have a positive supported birth in her new location, with her new provider.

In calling this the midwives model of care, these principles are framed around the shared practices of midwives, but doctors can also use this model. There are doctors who offer their clients everything detailed above, and occasionally midwives who do not. The model provides a unified alternative to a medicalized model of care, but that doesn't mean *all* midwives adhere to it or that *all* doctors practice a medicalized model.

DIFFERENT TYPES OF MIDWIVES IN THE US

As much as there is unity among midwives about the midwives model of care and the value of midwifery, the word "midwife" doesn't reference one type of education, training, credentialing, or practicing professional. It's confusing that the term "midwife" is an umbrella, but understanding this can help you navigate choosing if midwifery care is right for you and what type of midwife you'd like to work with. Below I detail a bit of history, not because the history itself will be valuable for you in your decision to work with a midwife, but because it's useful for understanding the *types* of midwives and how they differ.

Today approximately fifteen thousand midwives attend births in a wide variety of locations with very different skills, capacities, licensing, and legality throughout the country.[4] Historically, nearly all births were attended by midwives or traditional birth attendants until anti-midwife campaigns radically changed this. In the first half of the twentieth century, campaigns presented midwives as untrained, incompetent, and dangerous. Birth was seen as damaging and punishing, best managed by doctors with medications, surgical interventions like episiotomies, and clinical tools like forceps. Campaigns against midwifery and homebirth, and for obstetricians and hospitals, changed how people gave birth.

The rise of obstetrics in the US rapidly decreased the number of midwife-assisted births: only 10 percent of births were attended by midwives as of 1951.[5] This number would have been even lower, but poor women in the South lacked access to hospitals and obstetricians. Black midwives, often trained by their mothers, frequently called "granny midwives," continued to attend homebirths throughout the South even after the practice of midwifery was largely destroyed elsewhere.

The process of slowly rebuilding the number of midwives in this country and integrating midwives into hospital systems happened through multiple paths. One path was the Frontier Nursing Service, modeled after British nurse-midwives and established to aid poor families in Kentucky. Trained as nurses, these midwives largely attended homebirths until the 1950s when hospital-based midwifery programs were established. Today, 95 percent of certified nurse-midwives (CNMs) work in hospitals, with the remaining 5 percent split between homebirth and birth centers.[6] In my doula practice, I routinely work with CNMs who practice in hospitals and birth centers, as well as more than a dozen CNMs who attend homebirths in New York City.

In addition to nurse-midwives, informally trained "lay" or "direct-entry" midwives continued to attend homebirths. Some of these midwives were associated with religious and cultural groups, such as Amish midwives, and others became popular among white hippies in the 1960s and 1970s. One of the most famous midwives from that era, Ina May Gaskin, described to me attending her first births on buses in a traveling caravan, with no training other than a used obstetrics textbook and a belief that birth works. She's often credited with popularizing direct-entry midwifery in the US, although granny midwives deserve this credit, and has written a number of influential books about her experiences.

Most direct-entry midwives in the US today, including Gaskin, are certified professional midwives (CPMs), credentialed by the North American Registry of Midwives (NARM). This credential first became available in November 1994, establishing more standardized training, experience, and supervision requirements for direct-entry midwives, while still maintaining multiple paths into the midwifery profession. More than 2,500 CPM certifications have been issued since 1994.[7] CPMs provided support for out-of-hospital births, described by the NARM as "traditional, natural, non-interventive births."[8]

As mentioned above, midwifery laws in the US are a patchwork of state regulations (and lack of regulations). Only CNMs can legally work in all fifty states. CPMs, on the other hand, are nationally certified but must be licensed by the state(s) they want to practice in, resulting in fifty different sets of regulations, licensing boards (or lack of licensing board), and laws. One additional type of direct-entry midwife, certified midwives (CMs), take the same exams as CNMs and are officially recognized and able to practice in only a handful of states. There are also midwives practicing in the US who hold none of these credentials and are self-trained or traditionally trained in an apprentice model. Knowing the training and licensing of a midwife can be important because it could impact the care they offer (like the ability to prescribe medications or carry emergency medical supplies), their ability to bill your insurance for services, and what happens in the event transfer to a hospital is necessary.

One myth about midwifery care is that giving birth with a midwife is less safe than working with a doctor. Recent large-scale medical reviews have shown that having a midwife (a CNM or CM specifically) can result in better outcomes. For example, people being cared for by a midwife are less likely to have episiotomies and less likely to have larger perineal tears during delivery. They are also less likely to have labor induced and more likely to give birth vaginally. People who were randomly assigned to midwifery care also had fewer preterm births and fewer fetal losses, speaking to the quality of their prenatal care. Additionally, people cared for by midwives use fewer epidurals, report more satisfaction with their care, and have higher rates of chest/breastfeeding success.[9] Because 95 percent of CNMs practice in hospitals, this data largely reflects outcomes for people giving birth in hospitals.

Data on safety and outcomes with midwives outside of hospitals is limited. Writing about homebirth, the American College of Obstetricians and Gynecologists (ACOG) has said there are no adequate studies on planned homebirth, even from countries where homebirth is common.[10] At homebirths there are fewer interventions, which reflects the way midwives practice but also the choices made when planning a homebirth (e.g., epidurals aren't available at home so data confirming that epidural use is lower with planned homebirths is hardly surprising). Similarly, episiotomies, induction, and Cesarean births are lower, also not a surprise. We do know the safety of homebirth is increased by appropriate screening of candidates for homebirth and with the availability of timely transfer to a hospital if needed.

When Jesse gave birth to her daughter, she picked a CNM who offered homebirth services. The midwife told her she preferred to transfer to a hospital that was approximately an hour from Jesse's home (although there was a closer hospital they'd head to in an emergency). Labor was slow for Jesse, her water was broken for over a day, and she felt like pushing but was only 3 cm. Her midwife offered her options, including the option to transfer to the further away hospital for an epidural and rest. Devastated by this news and exhausted from days of labor, she made the choice to transfer. Hours later, after a long car ride and check-in process, an epidural, a nap, and an hour of pushing, Jesse's daughter was born with a hospital-based CNM. It wasn't Jesse's original plan—a tub in her living room without intervention or medication—but it remained a safe and positive experience with midwifery care, and she felt great about it.

The ACOG recommends carefully considering the type of midwife, especially when planning a homebirth. They've stated that CMs and CNMs meet or exceed the minimum criteria for education and training, but as many as two-thirds of CPMs do not.[11] Beyond training, because each state varies in how they license (or don't license) CPMs, there's huge variability in what medications or emergency treatments a midwife might provide. While a CNM anywhere in the US can carry IV fluids, medications to control postpartum bleeding, IV antibiotics, oxygen, vitamin K, and more, in some states CPMs can't carry any of these.

It's good to question your potential midwife about what they'll have and what they're comfortable using. While many people have advocated for uniform standards for midwifery care in the US, with all states adhering to a shared minimum requirement for education and training, until that happens, assessing the qualifications of a midwife, especially CPMs or uncertified midwives, falls to you.

HIGHER-RISK PREGNANCIES AND MIDWIFERY CARE

Midwives, on the whole, care for healthy people who are having uncomplicated, low-risk pregnancies. Initial screening can help sort out people who aren't a good candidate for midwifery care and should seek a doctor. Preexisting conditions like epilepsy or seizures, diabetes or a history of insulin dependent gestational diabetes, high blood pressure, bleeding disorders, or diseases like heart or liver disease, for example, might risk you out of midwifery care (especially if you were hoping to birth outside a hospital). Some things are considered higher risk but might have no impact on your access to midwifery care, such as being over thirty-five years old or using IVF. If you're considering midwifery care, speak to local midwives about your health and your history to see if they feel you're a good match for their services.

It's important to remember that even if you're a good match for midwifery care in the beginning of pregnancy, this can change. Reasons you might need to switch from a midwife to a doctor during pregnancy include a fetal health concern, like Terry's diagnosis of a fetal heart condition, or pregnancy-related health problems such as developing preeclampsia, cholestasis, or insulin dependent diabetes. All of these will likely make you too high risk for a birth center or homebirth, although a hospital-based CNM may continue your care, often with the assistance of an obstetrician. Additionally, going into labor prematurely or not going into labor before forty-two weeks can also risk you out of midwifery care, especially for planned out-of-hospital births. A breech baby, being pregnant with twins, and prior Cesarean birth or uterine surgery are also reasons some midwives (although not all) will risk you out.

When speaking with parents about their birth stories, I heard from several people who were considered by many to be too high risk to work with midwives but who'd given birth at home nonetheless. Sam, for example, planned a homebirth with a CNM, but her baby was breech and all efforts to move her daughter failed. Having exhausted all of her options for turning her baby, Sam said she could barely sleep thinking about what this meant for her birth:

> Our options were to schedule the C-section, pay over $15,000 for the one doctor in NYC who does breech vaginal deliveries (in a hospital nonetheless), or drive while in labor to upstate New York to a midwife who is known for doing breech deliveries. All of these options sounded terrible, so I called my midwife and begged her for the umpteenth time to allow me to have a breech home birth. In spite of her own fears and hesitation because of the legality of breech home delivery, she agreed. . . . We understood the risks associated with breech delivery and made an informed decision to move forward.

Shortly after getting her midwife to agree to assist with a breech homebirth, Sam began to feel mild cramping in her back followed by a big gush of water in the middle of the night. Labor was slow to start. She baked a cake, saw an acupuncturist to stimulate contractions, went to a diner for food, and walked laps on the roof deck of her apartment building as the sun was setting. Through all of that, the contractions became stronger and more frequent. Counterpressure on her back during the contractions and eventually laboring inside a tub helped her tremendously. By dawn she was fully dilated, and it felt good to push with contractions. She pushed first on a birth stool and later on her hands and knees in bed. She described her birth saying, "It was just so wonderful to have the breech home birth that I envisioned."

Similarly, Amaya chose to give birth at home with a midwife, even though she'd previously had a Cesarean birth and was higher risk because of it. She began her pregnancy looking for a doctor, researching VBAC rates and making appointments. Unfortunately, she "immediately disliked all of them" because "they all told me the same thing." Each doctor told her they'd support her in a trial of labor but "with the first sign of any complication I was going under the knife due to fear of uterine rupture." This felt too much like her previous birth.

With her first baby, Amaya worked with a hospital-based midwife but became aware of how limited her midwife's "power" was in the hospital. She recalled that as they wheeled her into the operating room, "my midwife turned to my husband and said that if the doctors had given me more time, I would have delivered the baby on my own. They were at the will of the hospital and had to walk on a very thin rope to stay in that hospital." Amaya felt that her first birth ended in an operating room because of a "knife-happy doctor and not because of any true emergency."

Amaya was most interested in a homebirth. Everything she read told her it was safe and might offer her the only real chance she'd have at giving birth the way she wanted to. She said, "A homebirth midwife would not have the constraints of a hospital system like my previous midwife had." She struggled to find a midwife who was willing to support a homebirth after a Cesarean birth (HBAC) but ultimately found one midwife who was open to talking. After they spoke, the midwife agreed to take Amaya on as a patient. Amaya described her care, saying:

> I could not have asked for a more caring, intelligent, strong and helpful midwife. She made the remaining months of my pregnancy happy. I didn't have to worry about my delivery because my midwife believed in my ability to birth my baby. She taught me to believe in myself too. She took such good care of my family,

helping all us feel comfortable and informed. The greatest gift she gave to me was finding my inner birth warrior. I was not afraid of how I was going to deliver the baby because I trusted my birth team and my body!

Describing her homebirth, Amaya said she had a "moment when time stood still and I experienced the true meaning of humanity. I delivered a human with only my body and my support team. It was a moment of pure power; pain (and exhaustion too) but pure power!" For her, the opportunity to be supported by a midwife in her home was transformative.

For Elle, being supported by midwives (and their backup doctors) in a hospital was the better option. Elle had given birth at home to her first child, and hoped for a second homebirth, but she was pregnant with twins. Elle's labor began with strong contractions and a gush of water. I joined her at her apartment while her husband took their daughter to a friend's house. We headed to the hospital where they confirmed both babies were head down and looking great on the monitors. She was already 5 cm, and everyone expected she'd give birth soon.

Although there'd been no sign of a problem at her prenatal appointment earlier in the day, Elle developed a severe case of preeclampsia during those short hours of labor. As she began to push, everything changed rapidly and she required all the emergency treatments a hospital has to offer. Working with a midwife in the hospital gave her immediate access to an operating room, surgeons, and emergency medical treatments, all things she needed.

Midwifery care is not appropriate for all pregnant people. Further, midwives practice in all birth locations, and determining which location makes sense for your birth is an important choice. For Amaya and Sam, they both felt giving birth with a midwife at home would give them the best chance of having the birth they wanted, even if they were higher risk. For Elle, seeking the care of midwives (and their backup doctors) in a hospital was a better choice.

Myths and misunderstandings about midwives lead many to believe doctors are their only choice, but a midwife can support you in the hospital or out of hospital, with pain medication or without. Midwives support a wide variety of healthy pregnant people and employ a model of care that emphasizes attention to your physical, psychological, and social well-being. Midwifery care can be nurturing and individualized, with a focus on education and support, and attention to minimizing interventions. Plus, there's excellent data on the safety of working with a midwife and on parents having positive feelings about their care. If giving birth with a midwife sounds like a good choice for you, find out who's available locally and what locations they work in.

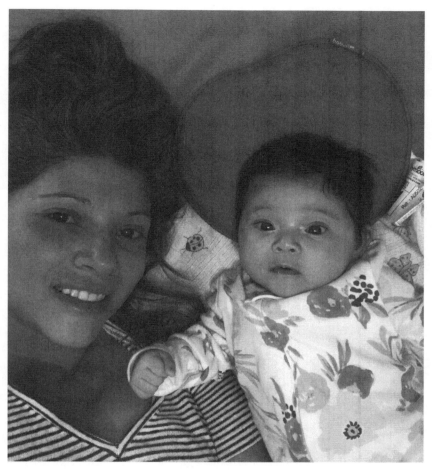

New mother and baby, supported in pregnancy and birth by midwives.

INTERVIEWING A HOSPITAL-BASED MIDWIFE

TRAINING AND EXPERIENCE

- What is your training/education/experience?
- How long have you been practicing?
- Do you offer any additional services personally or through your office that might be useful for me in pregnancy or postpartum?

HOSPITAL AFFILIATIONS

- What hospital are you affiliated with?
- If there are multiple, how much choice will I have in where I give birth?

COMMUNICATION

- Are you available twenty-four hours a day, seven days a week during my pregnancy?
- If not, when are you available and not available?
- How can I communicate with you during the pregnancy?

YOUR PRACTICE

- How many other care providers are in your practice? Are they doctors or midwives?
- Will I rotate between everyone in the practice for care or primarily see you?
- Will I have any choice over which provider is with me for the birth?
- Do you have residents, medical students, midwifery students, or nursing students assist you with my care during labor and birth?
- What tasks do they assist you with?
- What differences are there between the providers in your practice? What happens when you disagree with each other on the best approach?

SCREENING, RISK, AND TRANSFER

- What types of prenatal tests do you require? Recommend?
- How will you communicate the results of these tests with me?
- Are there circumstances that would require me to consult a doctor during pregnancy?
- Are there circumstances that would require me to consult a doctor during labor?
- Are there circumstances that would require transferring my care to a doctor?
- In the event of a transfer, are there doctors you would recommend I transfer to? Do you have a transfer relationship with anyone already? Can I transfer to someone else if I would prefer?
- Are there circumstances where you have disagreed with a doctor about caring for a client or managing a labor? What happens in those circumstances?

INDUCTION (ALSO SEE CHAPTER 11)

- Beyond more emergent signs that an induction is necessary, at what point in my pregnancy would you recommend scheduling an induction?

- How common are inductions in your practice? What percent of your clients do you induce?
- What induction techniques do you routinely use?
- What induction medications are available at the hospital where you practice?
- Will you be able to remain my care provider through all aspects of an induction?

CESAREAN BIRTH (ALSO SEE CHAPTER 14)

- How common are Cesarean births in your practice?
- What percent of your clients have Cesarean births?
- Who will perform the Cesarean?
- Will you be in the operating room with me during a Cesarean birth? What will your role be?
- Are gentle or family-centered Cesarean birth options available to me?

LABOR SUPPORT AND CHILDBIRTH EDUCATION

- Do you work with doulas? Can you recommend some?
- Do you work with birth photographers?
- Do you recommend a childbirth class to prepare? Can you recommend one?

POSTPARTUM SUPPORT

- What kind of postpartum care do you offer?
- Do you have experience with supporting chest/breastfeeding?

PERSONALITY AND PHILOSOPHY

- Why did you become a midwife?
- What is your philosophy of birth?

BUSINESS

- Do you take insurance? What type of coverage should I expect?
- What has your previous experience been with insurance coverage?
- How much do you charge, and by what date would the full amount be due?
- Do you accept payment plans? What is your refund policy if we switch care providers?
- Beyond payment for your services, what else I should expect to have to pay for my birth?

INTERVIEWING A HOMEBIRTH MIDWIFE

If you're planning a homebirth (or considering one), you'll want to set up interviews with local homebirth midwives. You do not need to ask all of these questions necessarily—just those that are important to you as you make your decisions about where to give birth and with whom.

TRAINING AND EXPERIENCE

- What is your training/education/certification?
- How long have you been practicing?
- How many babies have you caught? At home? How many as the primary midwife?
- Are you trained in neonatal resuscitation?

SCREENING AND RISK

- What things would make me "high risk" and need to transfer care during pregnancy or labor?
- Do you continue to see clients with gestational diabetes?
- How far overdue can I go and still birth at home? Are there any requirements that I have an ultrasound or testing if I do go overdue in my pregnancy?

- Do you require specific tests during pregnancy? If so, which ones?

TRANSFER RELATIONSHIP

- Do you have a transfer relationship with a hospital and if so, which one? If not, what do you do in the event that a transfer is needed (both in labor and also prenatally)?
- Do you have a backup physician? Do I meet with them during the pregnancy?
- What care would you provide to me if a transfer were necessary?
- Under what circumstances would you transfer to the hospital (e.g., in labor, postpartum)?
- Under what less than ideal circumstances would you stay at home?
- What is your hospital transfer rate?

CLINICAL TOOLS

- What equipment and supplies do you bring to a birth?
- Do you monitor the baby? With what tools do you monitor and how often?
- Do you carry oxygen?
- Do you carry antihemorrhagic drugs with you to all births? Which ones to you bring?
- Are you able to suture the perineum if necessary?
- Do you feel confident in your ability to suture? How much experience do you have suturing?
- How bad would a tear need to be for you to feel it required a hospital transfer?

LABOR SUPPORT AND CHILDBIRTH EDUCATION

- At what point in my labor will you come to my home to assist with labor/birth?

- Do you support water birth? Do you provide a tub for water birth, or can you connect me with someone who does?
- Do you work with doulas? Can you recommend some?
- Do you work with birth photographers? Can you recommend some?
- Who comes with you to the birth? If that person is another midwife, how experienced are they?
- If that person is not another midwife, what qualifies them to be a birth assistant? Can I meet with them before the birth?
- Do you require a childbirth class to prepare for homebirth? Can you recommend one?

POSTPARTUM SUPPORT

- What kind of postpartum care do you offer?
- Do you have experience with supporting chest/breastfeeding? Will you be able to help me with any chest/breastfeeding problems? If I am not planning to chest/breastfeed, can you help me with feeding my baby?
- How long do you stay after the birth? Do you help clean up?
- Do you provide postpartum visits in the days after the homebirth?

PERSONALITY, PHILOSOPHY, PRACTICE

- Why did you become a midwife?
- What is your personal philosophy of birth?
- How many births do you take on per month/year?
- Are you available twenty-four hours a day, seven days a week during my pregnancy?
- If not, when are you not available?
- How can I communicate with you during the pregnancy? Do you have a preference for phone calls, emails, or messaging?
- Who is your backup in the event that you cannot attend the birth?
- What is your experience with herbs, homeopathy, and alternative medicine?

BUSINESS

- Do you take insurance? What type of coverage should I expect?
- What has your previous experience been with insurance coverage? What about coverage in the event of a hospital transfer?
- How much do you charge, and by what date would the full amount be due?
- Do you accept payment plans? What is your refund policy if we switch care providers?
- What is included in the fees? What do I need to provide for a homebirth?

7

DOULA SUPPORT

I spent many years in college reading and watching cultural anthropologist Margaret Mead's books and movies. She focused on topics such as sex, gender, marriage, sexuality, child rearing, and parenting. As an undergraduate in New Mexico, I watched her old black-and-white films, fascinated by the images and Mead's narration of feeding or bathing babies in different cultures. Her cross-cultural studies remind us there are many correct ways to do things, and I embrace those messages in my mothering and as a doula.

One of the students Mead trained was medical anthropologist Dana Raphael, who coined the term "doula" to refer to nonmedical caregivers assisting during birth and the postpartum period. In *The Tender Gift: Breastfeeding*, Raphael wrote about her struggles to feed her son and how devastated she was by the lack of support she received. Raphael suggested new parents needed people to teach, support, and assist them as they learned to care for their babies (and themselves). She suggested this support was more about helping parents feel happy and confident than about the specifics of their choices, like breastfeeding or bottle-feeding.[1] As a young anthropologist profoundly changed by my own mothering experience, I loved following in Mead's and Raphael's tradition as I became a doula. In what follows, I describe what doulas do, why that work is important, and how to approach finding a doula.

WHAT IS A DOULA? WHY ARE DOULAS IMPORTANT?

When people ask me what I do for a living, I often choose not to use the word "doula" to describe my work, telling them I "help people have babies." For many, the term "doula" is unfamiliar, a meaningless term that tends to provoke a description from me and ends with the question: "So, you're a midwife?" I explain that doulas are not midwives, although there are places where our care for pregnant people overlap. Rather, a doula is a birth support person who provides continuous physical, emotional, and informational support during pregnancy, labor, birth, and the postpartum period. Unlike midwives, who perform clinical tasks, doulas are nonmedical professionals who aim to reduce fear, build confidence, increase knowledge, help with informed decision-making, offer practical support to cope, and serve as an advocate during labor and birth. I do these things with the primary goal of helping people have a positive experience of their birth—one where they feel informed and heard, respected and cared for, safe and supported.

As a doula I've taken on a wide variety of support roles in people's pregnancies and births. I've comforted and massaged, helped hundreds of people breathe through contractions, held hands during the scary or tough parts, and cleaned up vomit, blood, amniotic fluid, and more. I've held people while they cried, and I've laughed with them during funny moments. I have assisted people in laboring at home through hours of contractions, navigated hundreds of interactions with cab drivers as they transported my laboring client to the hospital or birth center, set up birth tubs, spoken with other members of their birth team or families, and advocated for them with hospital staff. I've stopped people from getting the wrong medications, noticed errors in care, helped clients avoid unwanted Cesarean births, noted symptoms that turned out to be significant, helped transport my clients from a homebirth to the hospital in a cab and an ambulance, and made sure my clients were able to communicate necessary information to their providers accurately.

I've made a midnight ice cream run for a laboring person who couldn't stomach much but thought ice cream might help. I've taken an old dog for a walk when a client didn't want to be separated from her husband and religious restrictions meant no one else they knew was available. I've helped more than twelve hundred people feed their babies through challenges and triumphs. I've wiped tears, given pep talks, helped people mourn, answered thousands of middle of the night texts and calls, prepared meals, and much more. I'm committed to helping clients in whatever ways they need. This is the type of flexible support from an expert in birth you might want and need during your birth (and beyond).

In offering this type of support, doulas not only help people feel better about their experiences of becoming parents, they also significantly increase the health and well-being of the families they work with. Dr. John Kennell, one of the first scientists to research the benefits of doula support, said, "If a doula were a drug, it would be unethical not to use it."[2] It would be unethical not to use it because decades of research have repeatedly affirmed the enormous benefit of having doulas present.[3] The improvements with doulas include increased rates of vaginal births and decreased numbers of Cesarean births, overall shorter labors, less use of Pitocin, less use of pain medication, less use of vacuums and forceps, higher Apgar scores at birth (an assessment of newborn health), and more success in chest/breastfeeding. Additionally, parents with doulas report more positive feelings about themselves and their infants. This is not to say that doula support is only for people who want vaginal births, would like to avoid pain medication, or are planning to chest/breastfeed, but to say that doulas can help people avoid unnecessary or unwanted interventions (while advocating for whatever you'd prefer).

When I asked doulas about what they thought accounted for these clinical improvements, they offered a wide variety of insights.[4] Prenatally, doulas help clients feel calm, confident, and capable in their bodies; they provide evidence-based information and educate their clients about pregnancy and birth; they assist clients in articulating their preferences, facilitating their search for a provider and birth location that matches their hopes and plans, and encouraging them to make the best decisions for themselves throughout their experience. Doulas also routinely move between different hospitals and birth centers, working with a wide range of providers, and this affords them a unique perspective they can share with clients as they plan for their birth.

The doulas I spoke to emphasized the importance of doulas' continuous support during labor. Doulas typically join clients in their home in labor and support them well before they might head to a hospital or birth center or see their doctor or midwife. This means doulas routinely see more of labor than other birth workers, and this perspective affords doulas a unique expertise in birth. Additionally, your doula should be focused on your care alone, unlike many hospital-based care providers who might have multiple patients in labor at once. Further, clinical providers typically have lots of paperwork and responsibilities to the hospital or birth center where they work while your doula can be present for you. Having a doula with you can help make more space for you to ask questions, to have things explained more thoroughly, to explore your options, and to make the right choices for you.

As a doula, I don't care what choices you make. I'm not being callous, quite the contrary. I think this is an important attitude for a doula. Your choices are your choices, never mine (or anyone else's), and my goal is to help you make choices you feel good about. My investment is never in the specific decisions you make. Rather, I care about assisting you in making decisions that are right for you. I help people formulate questions to ask as they gather the information they need. I help people think through the pros and cons (and alternatives) as they make their choices. A doula's support should be unconditional and without judgment, ensuring that you have the best possible experience you can have—whatever that means for you.

When I asked new parents about how their doulas had improved their birth experiences, their responses ranged from specific forms of assistance to more generalized praise. Specific physical support roles such as help with breathing, massage and touch, and positioning were commonly mentioned alongside emotional and educational support. Some responses were more humorous, such as the person who wrote back, "Um yeah, she was like an angel who saved my life and my sanity. No big deal." Others were more serious: "She kept me calm, sane, and reminded me that I could do it. She remained present, offered hands on relief as needed and when push came to shove (literally), she was there to get my doctor and help bring babe into the world." One person said her doula was really "valuable in understanding the helplessness and exhaustion my partner was experiencing." She noted that "so much" of her own "stress and anticipation was wrapped up in how he would cope," so when her doula encouraged her partner to take breaks to nap and eat, this was valuable. Another person told me her doula helped her hand-express colostrum, the first chest/breast milk, so her baby could be fed her milk even when the baby needed care in a NICU. Others said their doulas advocated for them with nurses, doctors, and midwives when their needs were not being met or their voices were not being heard.

Francesca's story highlighted her doula's role as an advocate. She told me that in labor, when complications arose, her doula really helped turn things around:

> Our doula walked into an incredibly tense scene with me crying and staring off into space. The doctor and nurse were telling me over and over again that a c-section might be necessary. Minutes before she got there, my baby's heart rate had dropped considerably during a contraction and the doctor freaked out on me. My area of expertise is technology and I know technology is not perfect. I could feel that my baby was not in danger and I wanted space to labor.
>
> I felt like the doctor and nurse went into panic mode when his heart rate went down. The nurse kept saying "this is bad" and "this is really concerning" in a tag team with the doctor. I asked if I could change position to see if that resolved the issue but they could not even hear me. The doctor kept saying to me that if the baby could not handle the contractions, I would need a c-section. It felt like they'd made up their minds.

When my doula arrived, she quickly read the scene and knew everything had changed in the few minutes since we spoke with her last. She gathered a little information and then came over and knelt in front of me. She talked to me in a way I could understand and accept. I knew she was in my corner and that she would help me get only the absolutely necessary interventions. She changed the whole dynamic in the room and I am certain that would not have been possible without her. I was being stubborn, the doctor was being stubborn, and communication was totally shutting down. Our doula spoke with the doctor and helped negotiate on my behalf. She defused the situation and brokered a plan both the doctor and I could agree to. I felt voiceless but my doula helped give me voice.

As much as the hospital and doctors are willing to help you or be less-interventionist, they are trained to do things differently. Ultimately, that's what they do. They intervene, they speed things up, and they help you the best way they know how but for me, that's not my way. They own that space and deliver babies there all the time. It is their world and it felt like a battle to do things differently. My doula was a translator. They were bulldozing over me because I could not negotiate on their terms but my doula could speak their language and this helped tremendously.

Being a translator or a bridge were common phrases I heard when interviewing both parents and doulas, and this role, as Francesca's experience exemplifies, can be incredibly valuable. Doulas can help clients gather information so they can make better choices, leading to improved outcomes. Doulas can help clients negotiate plans and communicate with their team more effectively. And, unlike drugs, doulas have no reported adverse side effects.

The American College of Obstetricians and Gynecologists and the Society for Maternal-Fetal Medicine issued a statement in 2014 reporting that one of the most effective tools for improving labor and birth outcomes was the continuous support of a doula.[5] With only about 6 percent of the population currently using doulas for their births,[6] they argue this is an underutilized resource. I agree. This is not to say everyone should want or choose to have a doula—I haven't abandoned my commitment to people making their own choices. That said, I do believe that substantially more than 6 percent of the population would benefit tremendously from doula support.

Current major obstacles to greater usage of doulas include economics, availability, and knowledge about doulas. Doulas are rarely covered by insurance: it's usually an out-of-pocket expense for most people (unless you have access to and qualify for some of the subsidized low-cost and free community doula programs around the country). Fees vary enormously, often based on experience and geography, which can make access to doula care very affordable for some and cost prohibitive for others. Additionally, there are rural areas where few, or no, doulas are available, and many people in places where doulas are available are not aware of the work doulas do and therefore haven't considered the value of adding a doula to their team.

HAVING A DOULA ON YOUR BIRTH TEAM

Each year I have about fifty interviews with prospective clients looking to hire a doula for their birth. I typically go to people's homes for these meetings, talking in their living room or at their table. Sometimes the meeting feels more formal—they have a list of questions prepared and ask me each one, weighing my answers against what they want for their birth. Other times these meetings are incredibly intimate with potential clients immediately entering into the doula relationship, disclosing a history of rape to make sure I can support them if this trauma becomes a factor in their birth, or recounting the sadness of terminating a wanted pregnancy after devastating test results made clear the pregnancy should not continue. The meetings are as varied as my clients, but my goal is always to meet people where they are, whether that means being present with tears and trauma or talking through questions as they gather information about me, about doulas, and about what to expect in their birth.

Prospective clients are often curious how I (or any doula) will work with the rest of their birth team: their husband, wife, partner, family, friends, midwife, doctor, and/or nurses. They wonder how I negotiate advocating for them without being adversarial or creating conflict with their provider. They want to know how I might comfort and care for them in such an intimate and intense moment without edging out their partner or other support people in the process. These questions are important. There are unfortunate stories of people who had disappointing experiences with their doulas—who felt their doula created a hostile environment by arguing with the staff or who behaved strangely with their family and friends in a way that did not make for a positive experience. These are exceptions, though, and not common. The interview is important to help you see if the doula you're considering is a good match for your personality.

Sometimes the client I'm meeting with already had a doula for a previous birth and is seeking something different in their doula care this time. Similarly, previous clients of mine have hired other doulas for subsequent births. This, of course, saddens me and makes me reflect on our interactions—how could I have done better, been more present or attentive, read their needs or desires more accurately? Yet I understand that the doula relationship is personal and things like chemistry, rapport, and finding a good match are as important, if not more important, than the value added by a doula's training, qualifications, or experience.

The world is full of lovely people whom you might nevertheless not pick to be your care provider or your friend because they're not a good match for your personality and preferences. This is equally true when picking a doula. It's important to find someone who fits with your personality, who has a style of communicating you enjoy, and who has a philosophy about birth and doula work that matches your expectations and desires. Noa described the qualities she and her husband were seeking when they looked for a doula:

> We were looking for someone who was knowledgeable, who referred to research and best practices and knew her stuff, who was willing to guide us and advocate for us with doctors and hospital staff; we were looking for someone who was a good listener, who was flexible and open to whatever birth we might eventually have; we wanted someone who had a kind, grounded energy; and finally, we wanted someone with a good sense of humor.

Finding someone with the right match of expertise and personality is key. I have heard doulas critiqued as "crunchier-than-thou" and clients have told me they expected I would be "hippie-dippie" or not very smart. Theresa read a lot of doula websites in her search and felt many were "really pushy" in their framing of "unmedicated childbirth as the right way to give birth." That wasn't for her, so she found someone with "a more open-minded approach." Tammy told me she read reviews and websites looking for someone experienced, "no reiki, no crystals." She wanted someone practical and grounded who would not "shame me—even inadvertently. Non-judgmental was critical." Annie said that hiring a doula who was "super confident" made them feel more confident. In your own search for a doula, you should find someone you feel a connection to, whether that's someone "crunchy" or not, who has a communication style that matches your own, and who makes you feel calm and supported.

It's also important to ask about your doula's approach to supporting clients in terms of their flexibility, availability, and expectations about the limits to services. Can you contact them anytime with questions or concerns, and when should you expect a reply? When will they join you in labor, and what criteria do they use to determine that? Are there types of things they cannot or will not do for you, and if so, what?

Further, making sure that your own expectations of what a doula can (and cannot) do for you are reasonable and realistic is also important. A few years ago a woman called me seeking doula services, explaining that she wanted to hire a doula for an unmedicated childbirth. One of the most important things to her was that her doula would ensure that under no circumstances she'd be given Pitocin while in the hospital. I explained to her that while I could happily support her in her birth, no doula could (or should) make that promise. In addition to being used to induce or augment labor, Pitocin is also used to prevent and treat hemorrhages. While a doula could help her communicate her concerns and preferences with her provider, ultimately no doula has the power to prevent a medication from being used.

Similarly, I've had potential clients explain doula services as a kind of insurance policy against bad things happening in their births. While a doula can help you understand your options as you navigate decision-making and consent and can offer physical and emotional support throughout the experience, a doula cannot guarantee a specific kind of birth or outcome, nor can a doula prevent complications or the need for an intervention. Doulas reduce the likelihood of unnecessary interventions, but no one can entirely curb the unpredictability of birth. Being clear about what doula services will look like and what you can reasonably expect from the experience of having a doula is critical when adding a doula to your birth team.

Another important area where you should have a shared sense of expectations with your doula is what it means to be on call to attend your birth. The majority of doulas are solo practitioners who are working under incredibly unpredictable circumstances. Being on call twenty-four hours a day, seven days a week, means missing holidays, special events, kids' recitals, and dinner with friends, and always being prepared to drop everything and run out at a moment's notice. For me this has meant not drinking, not seeing a show in a theater with bad cell reception, not traveling more than about forty-five minutes from my home, and always having child care available at a moment's notice. Being available like this for another person is no small commitment to make. There are a few weeks around the estimated due date when babies are most likely to arrive, but babies also routinely come earlier (or later) than expected, and this should be factored in.

When will your doula be available, and what does that mean? How far away from your home might they be on the day you go into labor? How soon could you reasonably expect them to arrive to join you? If your baby comes earlier than expected, might they be out of town or unavailable, and if so, is there a backup plan in place for that time period?

Even when babies arrive in the general window around their estimated due date, it's also always possible your doula is at another birth. Unless your doula only takes one client every few months (not likely if they actively work as a doula), there's always a possibility two clients could have a baby at the same time. In my own practice this has happened to me about 2–3 percent of the time, and in those scenarios I send a competent, compassionate backup doula to support my client until I can join them. I'd love to be able to ensure that it never happens, but the best any doula can do is work hard to keep the probability of an overlap as low as possible while adequately preparing clients for the possibility and having backup available.

When interviewing a doula, you should also be aware that training and certification varies enormously and doesn't necessarily guarantee anything about an individual doula's level of expertise, professionalism, or qualification. There is no licensing process, and certification is totally optional. This is very different from many other professions, such as a doctor or nurse, a lawyer, an accountant, a massage therapist, or a plumber, among others. The current field of doula training options is a bit like the Wild West—there are no rules or requirements, anyone can call themselves a doula trainer, and anyone can print out certifications. In practice, it's largely well-established local, national, and international organizations (nearly one hundred of them) with experienced, well-respected doulas training new doulas, but consumers should understand there are currently no occupation-wide standards for what it means to be trained or certified as a doula. This is another place where the interview process is important. You can ask specific questions about training and experience to see if the doula you're interviewing is right for you.

Having said all of this about the possible pitfalls and things to be aware of when hiring a doula, I still absolutely believe that adding a doula to your birth team is something you should consider. Doulas are currently an underutilized resource, and all the data tells us they can be incredibly effective in helping you have a safe and positive birth experience. An experienced doula is an expert in birth with an expertise that is largely unique to our labor support practices. Hiring a great doctor you love or working with trusted midwives at your local hospital, birth center, or at home is so important. Adding a doula to that team can make an enormous difference in your overall experience, helping you feel more cared for and supported.

Noa told me that before getting pregnant she'd heard about doulas, but "the whole thing seemed very unnecessary and very New York." After a number of unfavorable interactions with her care providers, she realized how difficult it was for her to advocate for herself, "to speak up or reach out with questions, concerns, confusions, and disagreements." She said she couldn't manage the situation herself in the ways she wanted because she lacked the medical knowledge and research on best practices, but also because she was "intimidated and scared." The process taught her what a doula could do and led her to hiring me for both of her births.

Your doula will work as part of your birth team, alongside your clinical and nonclinical support team, serving as your advocate without being adversarial. Doulas should be well versed in common interventions and complications associated with birth and capable of explaining them to you (along with your clinical team), potentially serving as a translator if the medical jargon doesn't make sense. They should be aware of possible alternatives and able to help you ask questions to ensure you make informed choices about your care. A doula should know labor support techniques and position changes to help decrease your need for interventions and increase your chances of having an uncomplicated birth, regardless of your choices around birth location or pain medication. Your doula should ideally work for you, not your provider or the hospital corporation; as such, their insights and information should be unbiased, without judgment, and focused on your needs.

When I was pregnant with our first son, I'd never heard of a doula and therefore never considered hiring one. We took a comprehensive childbirth education class recommended by our care providers, and we had what felt like a straightforward vision—I'd be in labor and my husband would be my support person. We'd been together for nine years at that point and had successfully negotiated many other adventures. This seemed like a reasonable, if intimidating, plan. In retrospect I think there was something naive and misguided about the lack of thought I put into what the experience of birth would be like for my husband. We were both so focused on what would be happening to me, how I would cope, and how my husband could support and comfort me that I think we forgot that birth would also be an intense experience for him.

After we'd labored alone together for a full day and night (with occasional nurses and midwives stopping in to say hello, adjust a monitor, or administer a test), my mother arrived from across the country. When we called her to let her know I was in labor, we both imagined she wouldn't make it until after I'd given birth. My labor stretched on long enough that she got there well before our son. When she arrived, we were both incredibly relieved to see her. An avid gardener and baker, my mother brought flowers, fresh bread, and homemade strawberry jam. The room was transformed by smells reminding me of home. She arrived with fresh energy, helping hands, and a heart filled with love. She held my hand, helped me breathe through contractions, rubbed my back, and gave my husband his first break in more than twenty-four hours. Later he told me in that brief moment he took for himself, he stepped out of the room and cried. He was overwhelmed and exhausted, and it was really tough to see me in pain. Plus, he was about to become a father, arguably one of the biggest experiences of his life.

Hearing this story a few days after I gave birth, I hugged him and thanked him for how supportive he'd been during labor. While birth was obviously challenging for me—labor was the hardest thing I had ever done—it was not easy to watch the person you love go through that and not have the ability to fix it. I began to wonder about what birth support could look like. This is the path that led me to discovering Dana Raphael and the concept of doulas. And now, when I work with families, I am keenly aware of the insight I gained from my experience. I want couples and families to come through birth together feeling connected, supported, loving, and present with each other. I believe that my expertise, my ability to normalize birth, and my guidance with potentially stressful decisions (like when to go to the hospital or what to do when plans change) help them have that. I often explain to clients that their partner/family/friends (depending on who is invited) knows them—their likes and dislikes, their stories, their bodies—and I know birth. My knowledge of birth can help their other support people be present for them and do the things they already do well: be their person. Having a doula doesn't take away from the experience of birthing with your partner/people; it enhances it.

Aviv told me she hired doulas for all five of her births because she knew she needed touch and support, and her husband wasn't the person to provide that. She said, "My husband is nervous when he sees me in pain. It is tough for him, and I totally understand that, but I needed to have someone next to me who was not nervous. I needed someone who could be confident and calm to help me with the unknowns so I could feel empowered in my births." The support of doulas improved the experience of childbirth for her and her husband—giving her the support she wanted and needed and calming her husband in the process.

What you want and need in your birth will be specific to you. Building your birth team is an area where you have a lot of control and can make choices that fit your desires. As a doula myself, I claim no neutrality on the importance of doulas—I think everyone who wants a doula should be able to have one! That said, I also believe that childbirth is different for each of us and finding what works for you might mean having the support of a doula, a spouse or partner, and/or family or friends, or it could mean choosing to not have any of those types of support. As you imagine your birth, think about what will make you the most confident, what will help you cope, and how you'll navigate getting information and making decisions. If it feels like a doula might be a useful addition to your birth team, start researching local options by asking local friends, other new parents, care providers, and childbirth educators who they recommend; read online reviews and check out doulas' bios on their websites or elsewhere; and reach out to people who appeal to you to find out about availability, cost, and the possibility of an interview.

CHAPTER 7

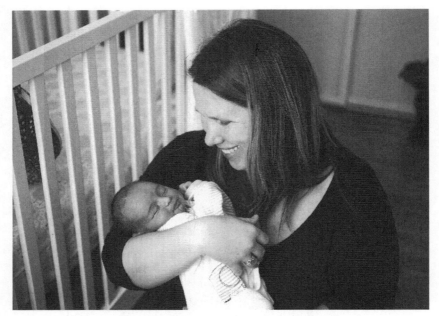

At a postpartum visit holding my client's baby.

INTERVIEWING A DOULA

If you'd like to hire a doula, you might start with some online research and then follow up over email or on the phone with anyone you're interested in knowing more about. Most doulas offer a free in-person meeting where you can ask questions and get to know each other. You don't need to ask all these questions—just those that help you as you make decisions.

- Why did you become a doula? (This question is often helpful in getting to know the person you are interviewing, their motivations for supporting people during childbirth, and their general philosophy about birth.)
- Can you tell me more about your training and experience?
- How many births have you attended? What's your experience with my birth location? Have you worked with the providers I've chosen or I am considering? Or, can you recommend birth locations or providers based on what our preferences are?
- Do you have experience with the type of birth I'm having (VBAC, the birth of twins, a homebirth, a higher-risk pregnancy, a planned Cesarean birth, etc.)? Have you worked with other clients like me or families like ours (single parents, surrogates, queer/trans families, bilingual families, families with religious traditions and restrictions, people of color, fat/plus-sized pregnant people, differently abled pregnant people, etc.)?

- How do you support laboring people during childbirth? Do you have special techniques or training you use? Can you describe what your support would look like for me? For my partner? For other support people who might be present? What does your support look like if I have pain medication? Or a Cesarean birth?
- How do you work with my doctor or midwife? How do you work with the nurses (if applicable to your birth location)? Or birth assistant?
- Can I contact you with questions? When? How often? Via what methods? How often do we talk? How often do we meet? What do we cover in those meetings?
- Do you have backup doulas available in case you can't be with us during the birth? Under what circumstances do you use backup? How often does this happen? Can we meet with or speak to your backup?
- When are you on call for me? What happens if I give birth outside that window? Are there times when you won't be available?
- When will you join me in labor? Where will you join us—will you come to our home prior to going to the hospital or birth center, or do you meet us there? How long will you be with us after the birth?
- What's your fee? What does it include? Are there things not included in this fee? In the event of a long labor, does the fee increase? What about a short labor? What's your refund policy?
- Do you offer chest/breastfeeding and postpartum support? If so, how much support is available to me? Can you refer me to other sources of lactation and postpartum support? Can I continue to call or email you for postpartum support and if so, for how long?
- Do you offer any other services such as prenatal yoga, massage, childbirth preparation classes, placenta encapsulation, birth or newborn photography, and so forth?
- Can we speak with previous clients of yours? (You might also look for online reviews.)
- Finally, some questions for yourself: Do you like this doula? Do you trust them? Do you feel supported by them? As much as weighing experience, training, or services matters when selecting a doula, rapport and personality matter enormously too.

GIVING BIRTH

8

LABORING

Iknew almost nothing about birth when I became pregnant. I'd seen TV sitcom versions of birth—a big gush of water followed by fast and furious contractions, a mad dash to the hospital, lots of screaming, "You did this to me!," a doctor commanding, "PUSH!," and a baby arriving shortly after. I knew enough to know they'd gotten it wrong but not much more.

On the advice of our care providers (I imagine they saw how clueless I was!), I signed us up for a comprehensive childbirth education class. It was hosted in the playroom of a local church. We sat on the floor, surrounded by stuffed animals and alphabet blocks, while our teacher—a nurse, lactation consultant, and mom—walked us through everything we should know. She covered the signs and stages of labor, our emotional states during each phase, when to go to the hospital, breathing and massage techniques, and all the interventions that might be offered or needed. We had weekly homework, quizzes in class, and hours of practicing various scenarios. I found role-playing awkward (pretending to be in labor felt like a task for a skilled actor and not me), and the birth affirmations felt silly (would I really be comforted by being told my cervix was opening like a flower or that I was a goddess?), but I still appreciated her enormously.

This class, the books I read, and the information I gathered from my providers, friends, and family were all important for me in gaining a more accurate picture of what to expect. Labor would be much longer than the mad dashes seen on TV sitcoms. Labor might be really hard, but I probably wouldn't scream at my husband. Labor might be scary or overwhelming, but my baby and I would very likely make it to the other side safe and healthy.

The traditional model of labor taught by my childbirth educator and presented in most books proceeds by stages and is often mapped out like a board game with multiple paths (for epidurals or extra-challenging labors or an unplanned Cesarean birth) and a happy couple holding a baby at the finish line. It reminds me of the board game Life that my son is fond of.

While the traditional stages model has been updated recently, which I'll explain below, it's still basically the same understanding of labor. I find it unhelpful because it doesn't speak to the lived experience of labor. Labor often doesn't follow the stages as they're presented, and this can cause confusion, doubt, and increased fear. Instead, I present a decentralized model for thinking about signs and symptoms of labor. I'm not going to map it out for you, because my experience is that each labor ultimately has a different map.

CERVICAL EXAMS AND STAGES OF LABOR

It is easiest to understand labor when you can visualize the basic anatomy of a pregnancy and recognize how doctors and midwives measure change during labor. At the beginning of your pregnancy, the placenta implants to the wall of your uterus connecting to your blood supply, and an amniotic sac extends from the placenta creating the "bag of water" that your baby will grow inside of. At the bottom of your uterus, inside your vagina, there is an opening called the cervix. The cervix is what the baby passes through during a vaginal delivery. In a Cesarean birth, an incision is made in the uterus above the cervix, and the baby is birthed through that incision. The cervix is central to how labor is clinically measured.

Cervical dilation is measured by a provider during a cervical exam, along with effacement, fetal station, and fetal position. The information from an exam can include:

DILATION: This is an estimate of how open your cervix is. The results will range from 0 cm to 10 cm (which is fully dilated). This is the most frequently discussed piece of information gathered from a cervical exam. It is worth noting that providers use their fingers, not a measuring tool, to estimate this opening so results can vary between providers.

EFFACEMENT: Your provider can also estimate how thin your cervix is, described as a percentage ranging from 0 percent to 100 percent. Some providers will also use descriptive terms like: thick, tight, firm, starting to soften, soft, stretchy, buttery, or ripe. When your cervix is thin, it tends to open more easily, so having your cervix well effaced is a great sign of labor progress.

STATION: This is an estimate of where the presenting part of the baby (their head unless the baby is breech) is relative to the ischial spines inside of your pelvis. When the head is high, this number will be −3 or −2, as the head comes down it will be −1 or 0 station, and when the head is low it will be +1, +2, or +3. Descent into the pelvis is important, as it can help the cervix open and can shorten the time you spend pushing.

POSITION: This is an assessment that can be made by feeling the baby's skull during an internal exam or by feeling the position of the baby through your belly (or by looking with an ultrasound). If the baby is anterior, they are looking toward your butt, and if they are posterior, they are facing forward (also called sunny-side up). A transverse baby is looking toward one hip. It's usually easiest to give birth to an anterior baby, so you may want to encourage your baby to be anterior before labor or during labor by avoiding reclined seated positions in favor of sitting upright, sitting on a yoga ball, hands and knees, and lying on your side.

Internal exams are commonly performed by OBs (and less commonly by midwives) in the weeks prior to your due date, before labor has begun. This information might be useful to you if you're curious, but knowing this information typically doesn't change anything about your care or your birth. Sometimes doctors or midwives make predictions about when your baby will be born based on an exam, but the predictions are often wrong. For this reason, some providers don't offer routine internal exams, and some people choose to decline exams at prenatal visits. (Earlier in pregnancy, exams can be used to gather useful information if there are signs of preterm labor.)

During labor, most hospitals and many birth centers require an initial internal exam upon arrival. This information is used to make decisions about whether to admit someone or to send them home to labor more. These requirements vary from facility to facility and depend on the specific circumstances of your own pregnancy and health. Your provider should be able to let you know what the criteria for admittance will be during your own labor. Additionally, if your birth location has a policy about intermittent versus continuous fetal monitoring during early labor, active labor, and transition, this initial exam might be used to determine the type of monitoring required (explained in the next chapter).

My experience of being in labor, and also in my work as a doula, is that the information gathered from internal exams during labor can have big emotional consequences. Some people choose not to have this information shared with them because they're concerned about their emotional response. My own emotions were very impacted by knowing how dilated my cervix was—with my first labor, finding out I was only 2 cm dilated when I'd been working so hard for many hours was devastating. Many hours later, hearing I was 9 cm was amazing news and made me feel encouraged and optimistic. I recognized that this emotional roller coaster might not be helpful for me, but I also felt like I needed to know—my curiosity was strong!

For Nell, finding out her dilation during labor was challenging. She recalled:

> After laboring for 16 hours we were all wondering how much progress I'd made. The exam was hard, as lying on my back was still difficult. And the news was not good. I was only at 3 to 4 centimeters, closer to 4 but this seemed like dismal progress, at least to me, after so much work. My midwife gave us a pep talk and said this was pretty good progress, not unusual, and showed us the chart of what 1, 2, 3 . . . through 10 centimeters look like. Ten looks like a huge hole, as big around as a large orange. Four is like a half dollar coin. I couldn't believe I had so far to go.

I have, similarly, seen many clients really deflated by the results of an internal exam, even when the exam was a poor reflection of labor progress. The cervix doesn't open in a straightforward way. For example, even though 5 cm is "halfway" dilated, being 5 cm does not mean you're halfway through labor—you might actually be fourteen hours into a seventeen-hour labor. Many years ago, a client and I headed to the birth center when her contractions were very strong and frequent, but she was turned away because her cervix was only 2–3 cm open. Her OB said we should labor at home for at least four hours before returning, but she gave birth less than two hours later. The internal exam was a poor reflection of where she was in her labor.

Most expectant parents are taught that labor is a series of stages that you're likely to experience—prelabor, early labor, active labor, transition (collectively called the first stage), pushing and giving birth (called the second stage), and delivering the placenta (the third stage). These stages and substages are divided based on the centimeters dilated your cervix is. Historically that was described as: up until 3 cm is early labor, from 3 to 7 cm is the active phase of labor, transition begins at 7 cm, and at 10 cm (or fully dilated), you move into the second stage and begin to push.

When cervical dilation is used to define labor stages and progress, this can be confusing and frustrating. It's not uncommon for a doctor to say something like "when you are in labor" or "when labor begins" to reference the active stage of labor, despite the laboring person very clearly already having contractions and feeling "in labor." Erin, for example, told me she felt "totally crushed" when her doctor told her, between strong contractions, that she was not yet in labor and that this was the "easy stuff" before the "real work" began. She went from feeling like she was coping with labor well to feeling "out of control." Getting back to a place of "being inside the experience"—instead of in those numbers and the obstetric stages—took a lot of effort.

This type of experience has become even more common recently due to updates in how the stages of labor are defined. In 2014, it was recommended that doctors reimagine the stages of labor with active labor beginning at 6 cm. In this new model, early labor, also called the latent phase, is 0 to 6 cm. With this longer latent phase, active labor begins much later, at 6 cm, and transition is still from 7 to 10 cm (but largely collapsed into the category of active labor). Pushing remains at 10 cm.[1]

The rationale behind this change—an effort to reduce interventions and unnecessary Cesarean births—is great, but in practice it can be challenging for people in labor to make sense of clinical criteria that might not reflect their experience. These reimagined stages help decrease interventions and reduce the frequency of Cesarean births for "failure to progress" or stalled labor. That said, mapping the stages of labor in cervical dilation has never felt particularly useful in terms of helping people make sense of their own labor progress—and in those terms, these new criteria make even less sense. If labor does not start until active labor—at least 6 cm—then most people spend the vast majority of their labor "not in labor" (which might not be helpful to hear between contractions).

SIGNS AND SYMPTOMS

Every labor is different—no one can give you an accurate map of exactly what your experience will be like. I don't rely on the clinical mapping of labor in my own work with pregnant people, and I don't find it especially useful in making sense of what you might experience in your own birth. What I can share with you, after hundreds of births and thousands of birth stories, are the *common* signs, the sensations *most people* experience, and the feelings *often* felt during the process. You might never experience some of these signs or symptoms, or you might experience them "out of order" in your labor. Early in my first labor I suddenly had two-minute-apart contractions and shaky legs. These are often signs associated with the end of labor, and I worried labor might be moving fast. Fifteen minutes later the burst of contractions and shaking passed. I returned to a slower pace, and nearly twenty hours later I gave birth.

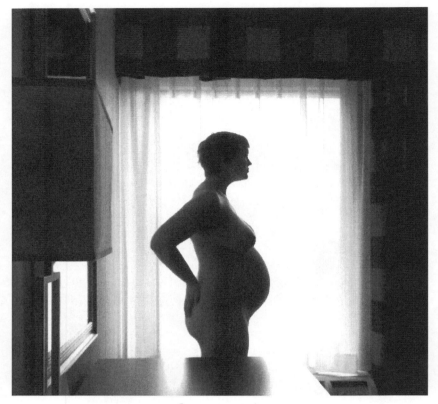

Pregnant portrait.

To move away from clinical stages of labor, I've instead organized this chapter around specific signs of prelabor and labor such as dropping or lightening, seeing your mucus plug, having contractions, the water breaking, bleeding, shaking and nausea or vomiting, frequent bowel movements, and rectal pressure. Following descriptions of each of these signs and how to interpret and manage them, I turn to descriptions of pushing, birthing your placenta, and the first hour postpartum.

DROPPING OR LIGHTENING

"Has the baby dropped yet?" I remember being asked this frequently by well-meaning strangers trying to strike up an awkward conversation about my body.

Often in the final weeks or month of pregnancy the baby will settle, or drop, into the pelvis. This can decrease pressure on your lungs and stomach, making it easier to breathe and eat, but the trade-off is often increased pressure on your bladder and even more trips to the bathroom. I really don't consider this a sign of labor at all; I include it here only reluctantly because there is much attention paid to lightening. When your baby drops—if they drop, some don't drop until labor—it's a normal part of the end of pregnancy and not a significant indicator or predictor of labor.

THE MUCUS PLUG

The consensus among people I know is that the mucus plug is among the more gross-sounding parts of labor. It has an important job, even if it could really use a new name. During pregnancy the cervix is typically long, tightly closed, and sealed with a thick mass of mucus blocking bacteria or infection from entering the cervix. That barrier stays in place throughout the pregnancy, but at some point—either prior to or during labor—the mucus comes out as the cervix thins and opens, making way for your baby to be born. If you notice mucus discharge earlier than a couple weeks before your due date, let your provider know.

When you're near your due date, noticing mucus discharge can be a good sign that your cervix is beginning to change in preparation for birth, *but* labor could still be anywhere from hours to weeks away. It can function like an early warning signal for some people. In Sarah's case, for example, it was an early sign that labor was beginning. She told me:

> I was about 6 days before my due date and we had a really busy day. We'd missed one of our childbirth ed classes and had a make-up scheduled, immediately followed by a newborn CPR class. The teacher in the CPR class joked that when people take the class that late in their pregnancy, they usually go into labor right away afterwards. I thought it was funny at the time but it turned out to be true.
>
> I was exhausted after both classes. I wanted to go see a movie because I thought I might not get to do that again for a long time (which is totally true because it's now two years later and I still haven't gone back to a movie theater!) but I was too tired. We went home, ordered pizza, and watched a movie on the couch instead.
>
> I went pee during the movie and I noticed my mucus plug had come out into my underwear. I wasn't having any contractions or other signs but I texted my doula to let her know. She said that this might mean the baby was coming soon or it could still be a couple weeks. We'd just have to wait and see.

> During the night I started to have a pain in my back that was spreading and washing over me. It felt like it came from the middle of the back and spread all around my sacrum. It was about 3am when that started and I knew it was labor beginning.

In Sarah's case, the mucus plug was a good indicator that things were beginning. For others, it might not indicate much. I've had clients lose parts of their mucus plug for weeks before labor, and this is normal. It's also normal to not notice any mucus prior to labor. If you notice small amounts of brown, pink, or red blood mixed with the mucus, this is also normal. If you've recently had a cervical exam or sex, both can cause cramping, discharge of mucus, and small amounts of bleeding—but this is not necessarily the beginning of labor.

CONTRACTIONS

When I was pregnant with August, my older son, I remember feeling intensely curious about what labor would be like. *How will I know I am in labor? What will it feel like? What if I don't know I am in labor?* I wanted to know exactly what a contraction would be like and how I'd recognize I was having one. I asked questions of my childbirth educator, I searched for clues in books, and quizzed my providers, friends, and my mom.

The answers were less helpful than I'd hoped. "Contractions start off like menstrual cramps," they told me. I was told that I would "know." This was a frustrating answer. And yet, after a few weeks of feeling all sorts of tightening, cramping, and strangely uncomfortable feelings, I woke up one afternoon from a nap and felt a strong wave of cramping discomfort very low in the front and wrapping around to my back. It reminded me of my period and also of what the warning signs of diarrhea might feel like. As quickly as it came, the sensation passed. Ten minutes later I felt it again. Everyone was right: I knew. (Although I should note, when I "knew" I was in labor the second time, I was wrong and did not give birth for another week!)

Some of the earliest signs of labor for most people are contractions—often mild or spaced out or a slowly building crampy feeling. In the beginning, contractions may be far apart and irregular, or they may be closer together and more regular immediately. It's also possible to have contractions on and off for days, sometimes even weeks, before labor begins (called prodromal labor). You might feel excited, anxious, happy, afraid, or uncertain—or all of the above! Sometimes contractions are triggered by exhaustion or dehydration; these contractions tend not to be the beginning of labor. Drinking lots of water (or other beverages) can be helpful. Eat if you're hungry because you might need calories to keep your energy up. For most people, ideal foods are high in protein and carbs but not too spicy or acidic (you may throw up later).

When contractions begin, some people find that walking can be helpful, especially if they feel restless or have a lot of anxious or excited energy. That said, if contractions begin during the night, it can also be great to stay in bed and sleep (or be sleeplike) for as long as possible. Be honest about your emotions, and find ways to rest and relax your body and mind. Shower, stretch, breathe, and talk to your birth team to let them know what's happening. Many people enjoy distraction—watching movies, reading, playing a game. Be aware that it is totally normal for contractions to begin and then stop—don't be discouraged.

When clients ask me how to identify labor, I talk to them about contractions coming in a progressive pattern—contractions becoming more frequent, stronger, and/or longer in length. If contractions start at ten minutes apart and move to seven minutes apart and then to five minutes apart, you're in a progressive pattern. If contractions start at four minutes apart and very mild but grow stronger, that would also be a progressive pattern. Most contractions ultimately become about a minute long (sometimes slightly longer or slightly less), so another index of a progressive pattern would be contractions that began as twenty- or thirty-second cramps and grow into sixty-second-long waves. If your contractions are irregular, infrequent, or don't seem to be changing in any progressive way, it might mean labor has not begun or more patience is needed. Our bodies are not machines, and the process is not always as predictable as the descriptions of it seem.

As contractions become progressively longer, stronger, or closer together, the feeling of pressure might also increase. Emotions might shift toward feeling more serious and focused, concerns about where you are in the process, fear and anxiety about what comes next, and happiness in knowing labor is happening are all possibilities, among others. More labor-coping strategies will likely be needed to manage the contractions. Being upright, on hands and knees, on a yoga ball, in the shower, or resting and breathing to relax are all nice options for laboring at this point. Vocalizing with the contractions ("ohhhh" or "aaahhh" or "uugghh" sounds), keeping your jaw relaxed, dropping your shoulders, and trying to clear your mind of worries or fears (or speaking them out loud) might be helpful. You may no longer feel like eating, but staying hydrated is important: drink often and try to urinate often.

Labor can continue like this for a long time or a relatively short time. Your doctor or midwife will likely give you some criteria for when they want to hear

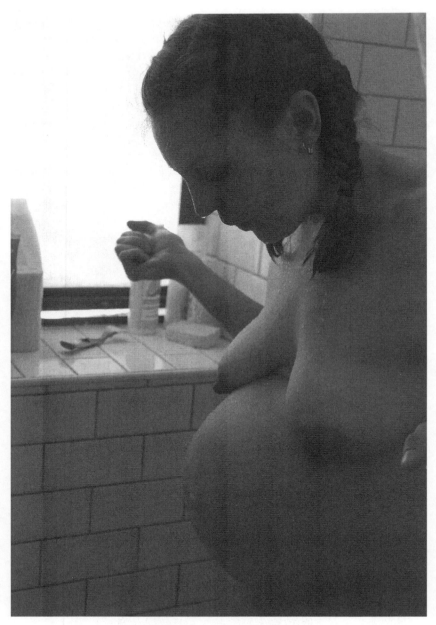

Laboring in the shower at home.

from you and when they want you to go to the hospital or birth center (or come to your home). These criteria often include bleeding (beyond spotting), water breaking, and frequent contractions. As labor progresses, the contractions will typically happen at least every five minutes and last at least one minute. When this has been going on for at least an hour, the pattern is called 5-1-1 (five minutes apart, one minute long, for one hour). The 5-1-1 pattern is often used by providers to help identify the beginning of active labor. If the contractions are more frequent, four minutes apart, it's called 4-1-1.

Your provider will likely tell you to call or come in based on patterns like these. With your first baby this will be at least a 5-1-1 pattern, often 4-1-1 or 3-1-1. Because first labors are, on average, longer than subsequent births, your provider will use different criteria if this is not your first birth. They'll likely recommend you reach out to them earlier and come to the hospital or birth center (or have your midwife come to your home) earlier. Additionally, your health and birth plan can influence when you should be contacting your provider and when they want to see you. For example, people who want epidurals usually go to the hospital earlier than those planning to avoid epidurals, and people who test positive for group beta strep (GBS) are seen earlier to make sure they get IV antibiotics (explained in the next chapter). Talk with your provider prenatally about when they'd like to hear from you in labor.

As labor grows more intense and contractions more frequent, many people feel more determined, less social, and have a greater need for a less stimulating environment. If you were watching a movie or playing a game, you may end up abandoning it to focus on labor. Again, more labor-coping strategies will be used to manage these contractions as the pattern progresses. Continued vocalization, keeping your jaw and shoulders relaxed, and taking a shower or a bath can be helpful. In upright positions, try to keep your feet planted on the ground with your legs hip width apart. If you want to move, rock side to side or bend your knees and dip into the contraction. Your instinct might be to move away from the pressure—pulling up or closing your legs—but moving *into* it can help the labor progress and reduce pain. Lying on your side with your legs open, especially around a peanut ball, can also be helpful.

For Lina, lying on her side through contractions worked well, and she recalled both how she managed the contractions and the shift she felt as she moved into pushing:

> The contractions soon became so painful that I couldn't bear to change positions anymore, so I stayed lying on my right side in the bed. Our doula was massaging my tailbone through all the contractions, and my husband stood by my head and I

held onto his hand, squeezing it ferociously during each contraction. I found that my doula's hands on my lower back were the perfect physical reminder of where to focus my breath. As each contraction began to rise in intensity, I focused on directing my breath, in and out, from where her hands were. I also experimented with sounds I could make that were low-sounding ("RRRrrrrrrr" and "oooohh-hhhhwwwww"). I had one minute to recuperate between each contraction, and I found I needed that minute to concentrate fully inside of myself. I couldn't open my eyes or talk to either my husband or doula—it was too distracting and offered way too much stimulation. I felt desperate to focus deeply and ground myself in those recovery minutes to prepare.

The contractions kept growing in intensity, and suddenly there was one that jumped up to a whole new level and I felt the baby moving downwards forcefully at the same time. I got scared for a second because it felt like things had shifted and I was now pushing the baby out without being able to control it. The doctor hadn't even arrived yet, and I had no idea how dilated I was so I was terrified that I might injure myself. It had only been about three hours that I'd been labor, but it felt like things were really progressing. Our doula was wonderfully calm and unfazed and confirmed that it looked like I had started pushing a bit. She talked me through a couple ways to breathe to avoid pushing on the next contractions and also calmly encouraged the nurse to bring the doctor, telling her that I'd been feeling the urge to push on the past couple contractions.

Finally the doctor arrived, did a quick check to see how dilated I was, and said, "oh yes! Are you ready to have this baby?" I was confused by her language, and a little furious. I HAD BEEN HAVING this baby for hours already! Of course, she just meant the baby was right there and I was dilated enough to start pushing.

In Lina's birth, breathing and vocalizing, massage, and squeezing her husband's hand were her primary coping strategies for getting through contractions.

Throughout labor, staying as calm as possible, being focused on the present, and feeling connected to your support people are important. Drink lots of fluids, eat small snacks if desired (some people don't want food, and this is also fine), use the bathroom frequently (having an empty bladder can help the contractions feel less intense), and remember to use the space between contractions to relax, as Lina described. If you don't have an epidural during this stage of labor, it's common to have increased self-doubt, fears that you cannot make it much longer, or a sense of defeat.

Many people will announce that they can't do it or begin thinking or asking about pain medications at this point. The pressure can be scary and overwhelming. I remember feeling like the baby was in my butt, and the sensation was both not what I expected and very intense. Remind yourself that you're safe. Your self-doubt can be a sign of progress and how near you are to the end of labor. It can be helpful to remember you'll soon be holding your baby (and labor will be over, whichever is more reassuring). For many people, managing contractions is an intense experience of surrendering both physically and mentally. I like to remind people that this is temporary, labor cannot go on forever, and to stay in the moment as much as possible.

When I helped Caroline have her baby, we arrived at the hospital and her doctor confirmed that she was 9 cm and the baby was very low. She was thrilled at the news that she was so close to having her baby but also overwhelmed by the intensity of the sensations. Between contractions she began saying to me, "Tell me something about this contraction." I would reply, "It's temporary." "Tell me something else," she would say. "It's getting you closer to your baby." She nodded. "Tell me something else." We made eye contact. "You can do this." She nodded again. "Ok, I can do this. It's temporary. I'm getting closer to meeting my baby." Then the next contraction began. Committed to laboring without an epidural, finding ways to be encouraged and to cope through the last couple of hours of labor was really critical for Caroline. What works for you might vary greatly from what work for other people (see chapter 10 for more on labor-coping strategies).

THE WATER BREAKING

The amniotic sac attached to your placenta fills with amniotic fluid early in pregnancy. This helps to cushion and protect the baby as well as assists in maintaining a consistent internal temperature, and it's used by the baby to practice using their digestive system and breathing. Most people are familiar with the concept of the "bag of water" because TV shows would have us believe that a big gush of water is always the first sign of labor. In truth, only occasionally does the water break before contractions begin. Your water might break at any point during the labor, or your provider might perform an artificial rupture of the membranes with a tool called an amniohook—a plastic wand (described in the next chapter). On more rare occasions, babies can also be born inside of their amniotic sac (in the caul) with the water only breaking after the head is out (like Paula's story in chapter 3).

Sometimes when the water breaks there is a sound, as Robin described: "I HEARD a distinct 'pop' sound, like . . . a cork popping. And then I felt a spreading wetness all around me." Other times, there is a feeling as the water breaks, such as Nina's experience. "I was on the couch eating a Chinese food lunch (pork fried rice, egg roll, chicken and broccoli) and watching an episode of the BBC show 'Call the Midwife' when my water broke. I felt something and got up from the couch and then a big gush followed." Nina laughed about her experience, describing it as "very authentically ME." Dee felt and heard her water breaking also. She told me, "I looked over at my husband and said, 'Did you just hear her kick me?' And then waterworks."

When the amniotic fluid releases, it is not a singular incident—you'll continue to leak amniotic fluid until your baby is born, with small gushes or trickles during contractions or periodically when you or the baby move. Farrah's water broke at home, but twelve hours later she was still not in labor, so she took a cab to the hospital for Pitocin to start labor. She recalled, "No one had warned me that the amniotic fluid keeps coming and coming and after the car ride and some walking I guess enough had shifted. It was as if I'd sprung another leak. I stood there in the hospital lobby in my summer dress, dripping everywhere, trying to look nonchalant and non-contagious as other people backed away and took a separate elevator."

Many of my clients have worried out loud about their baby after the water is released: Are they like a fish out of water now? While the baby is less cushioned and protected from infection once the sac has broken, there is still some fluid around the baby throughout labor and they're still getting oxygen and nutrients from the umbilical cord.

Sometimes when the water breaks it occurs as a big gush of water—Tara described it as Niagara Falls with water gushing out of her—but other times it is a slower leak with lots of smaller, consistent trickles of fluid. When Lina's water broke she thought it was urine. She said, "I woke up at 5am on Sunday needing to pee. Walking to the bathroom, I felt a trickle down my thigh and kind of groaned to myself, thinking, 'Oh great! A new pregnancy-related indignity to deal with: now I am peeing on myself!'" So many people imagine that it will be very obvious when the water breaks—and sometimes it is—but many of my clients are unsure. It's not uncommon to have an increase in discharge in the days and weeks before labor begins, and it's also not uncommon to leak urine in pregnancy. This additional wetness can prompt questions and confusion. If you have multiple trickles in a row, that's a better indication it might be your water. Check in with your provider if you think your water has broken.

Also, take note of the color and odor of the fluid. Amniotic fluid is usually clear, a little pink from mixing with small amounts of blood, or clear with mucus mixed in. If it smells like urine, it probably is; amniotic fluid doesn't smell like urine. If it has a yellow or green tint to it, your provider will want to know that. This discoloration can indicate that the baby has pooped (meconium) in utero, and your provider will likely want to monitor the baby to make sure this isn't a sign of stress. When you're further past your due date, the likelihood of there being meconium in your fluid increases.

After your water breaks, your provider will likely want to talk through a plan. If your water breaks when you're in labor, that's a good sign of labor progress. If contractions haven't begun yet but start within a few hours of the water breaking, most providers are also reassured. On some occasions, intervention is recommended to help contractions begin (see chapter 11 for more). When you test positive for GBS (discussed more in the next chapter), IV antibiotics are recommended as soon as the water breaks, and your provider might recommend medication to start contractions and minimize the time the baby is potentially exposed to GBS. Although having your water break prior to contractions is less common, it can be good to talk with your provider prior to labor about how they'll want to manage that situation. Ultimately the choices will be yours, but working with a team that has the same preferences you have is ideal.

BLEEDING

You might be concerned by the sight of blood, but it is not uncommon to have spotting during pregnancy (about one-third of people experience this) and it's incredibly normal to bleed a small amount during labor. Bleeding *prior* to labor should never be ignored, but it might not be concerning either. For example, as mentioned earlier, if you have recently had a cervical exam or sex, both can often cause a small amount of bleeding. Check in with your provider. In pregnancy you have significantly more blood than you did before pregnancy, and it's normal to have some bleeding during labor, a more significant amount of bleeding directly following the birth, and then several weeks of postpartum bleeding. Most bleeding during labor is spotting or small amounts of blood mixed with mucus. When you are getting closer to pushing, there is often a larger period-like amount of blood called the "bloody show," and this is a normal sign of labor progress.

SHAKING, NAUSEA, OR VOMITING

During labor it's common to experience some shaking. This shaking can be caused by hormonal shifts in your body, by adrenaline during intense moments, or by temperature changes during the hard work of labor. It's not uncommon for people to feel hot when they're having a contraction—throwing off blankets, wanting to be fanned or touched with a cold washcloth—but when the contraction passes, sometimes people start to shake and need to be covered and warmed. Other times the shaking has nothing to do with being cold, and a blanket will not help. For many people, shaking happens later in labor when the contractions are close together and you're getting closer to pushing, but it can happen at other points as well.

Feeling really nauseated, and sometimes actually vomiting, are also normal in labor and not a sign that anything is wrong. As a doula, I carry emesis bags, especially for the car ride to the hospital or birth center, but you might also find them useful if you experience a lot of nausea and vomiting in your pregnancy. Theresa recalled becoming really nauseous and throwing up a lot toward the end of her labor. She already had an epidural and couldn't leave the bed, but I'd brought "amazing space age barf bags." She said, "The hospital had nothing and I would have been throwing up everywhere without those bags. They are really the best possible thing!"

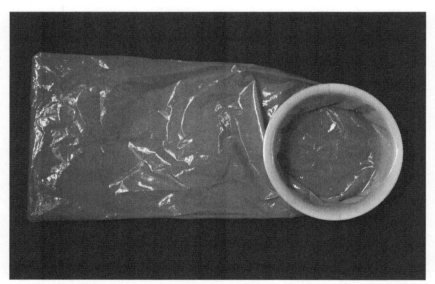

A vomit bag, easily available for purchase and great for pregnancy and labor.

Even though you might throw up, it's still OK to eat and drink to stay hydrated and to keep calories in you for energy. Ice cream is a great labor food because it is easy to eat and high in calories. If you find that the nausea and/or vomiting are preventing you from staying hydrated, communicate with your providers. IV fluids for hydration and IV medication to help prevent throwing up might be available and a good option.

FREQUENT BOWEL MOVEMENTS AND RECTAL PRESSURE

During the course of labor you might have frequent bowel movements. Often this can be an early sign of labor, and you'll likely feel increased pelvic pressure. As the baby moves lower, or if your bag of water is starting to bulge inside of you with contractions, you'll likely feel rectal pressure unrelated to actually needing to have a bowel movement. For this reason, some people describe their water breaking as a feeling of relief. Frequent bowel movements and rectal pressure can make the toilet a comfortable place for laboring—even if nothing comes, you might feel more relaxed knowing you have the option. That sensation is the baby's head low in your pelvis putting pressure on your rectum.

As the rectal pressure increases, you may feel yourself beginning to bear down or grunt during contractions. For some this is a gentle shift with pressure increasing slowly and small moments of pushing during some contractions. For other people, this process can feel more abrupt with the body moving quickly into strong pushing sensations. Even with an epidural, it is not uncommon for people to begin feeling this pressure, and you should let your nurse or care provider know what you are feeling. Many providers like to perform internal exams to make sure your cervix is fully dilated when you begin to have an urge to bear down because that sensation occasionally comes before the cervix is fully open. If your cervix is not yet fully open, they'll recommend you try not to push, and it can be helpful to change positions and blow or pant during contractions to lessen the urge to bear down.

The transition from labor to pushing is usually marked with increased rectal pressure and the beginning of an urge to push. Years ago I read someone describing this moment as the time when you "thread the needle." This description makes sense to me—you have to go into the intensity of labor in order to come out the other side. If you are not already at the place where you will be giving birth and you are feeling rectal pressure, you should definitely be heading there. Again, being upright, on hands and knees, in the shower or bath, or lying on your side might be helpful. Vocalizing with low, slow moaning sounds can help you keep breathing slowly through the big feelings. As you keep yourself open (your jaw, your legs), you may begin to feel your body pushing involuntarily during contractions.

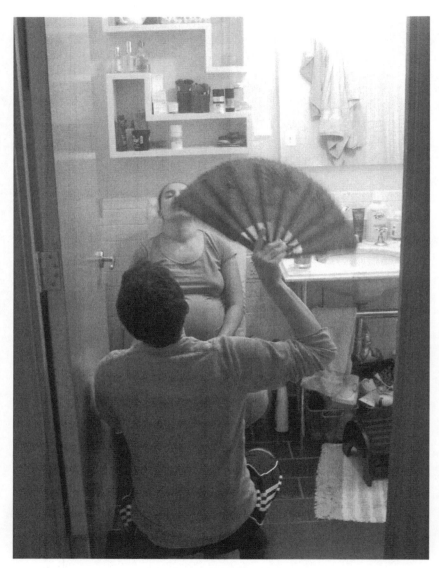

Laboring on the toilet at home.

PUSHING

With my first birth, the transition to pushing felt slow—too slow—and I was impatient for the labor to be over. It was hard to pant and blow and moan through the last couple of centimeters of cervical dilation before pushing him out. With my second son, the urge to push came on as a sudden sensation of "throwing down" (an intense involuntary feeling like throwing up but in a downward motion, pushing the baby out). When Jenny told me about the birth of her first child, she recalled her final pushes, saying, "The doctor asked me to stop for a minute so he could put on a gown, but that wasn't possible. My body was just doing it, the pushing felt involuntary."

It's not uncommon for clients to worry that pushing will be the hardest part of labor, but my experience has been that many (although not all) people actually prefer pushing. Perhaps this is because the end is in sight or because pushing is active compared to the more passive feeling of coping with contractions.

Many people have heard that they will poop while giving birth. It's true, you might. This sounds pretty mortifying to many of us, but the body often clears everything out during labor with lots of trips to the bathroom so if it happens, it will quite often be in the smallest, least significant amount. And for your provider this will be a good sign that you are pushing well.

In hospitals, it's common for nurses and doctors to coach you during pushing. This works well for many people, especially those who have an epidural. This coaching is often done in a semi-inclined position on the bed with your legs supported by members of your birth team. You'll usually be asked to put your hands behind your knees to pull your legs open and back during each contraction. Take a breath and hold the breath in, pushing down as though having a bowel movement. Often while you're holding your breath and pushing, your doctor or nurse will count to ten. This sequence is usually repeated three times per contraction.

If you find that holding your breath does not work well for you, it might be helpful to know that studies have not shown any significant benefit to pushing this way. As well, there is no evidence that coached pushing in general has any benefit over having laboring people bear down and push according to their own instincts, as a response to the contractions and pressure from the head coming down.[2] If you have an epidural and find you cannot feel enough sensation to push without coaching, one option is to lower or turn off the epidural to help you regain some sensation (although some people are not interested in this option at all).

Pushing in other positions can be beneficial, such as on hands and knees, on your side, squatting, or while standing. Some people find they push better while exhaling out or making noise, or pushing for shorter times than the suggested ten-count. Experimenting to see what works best for you can be helpful. If you don't have an epidural (and even sometimes when you do) you'll likely have an overwhelming urge to push and be guided by your own instincts. As with all of labor, this can be a quick stage (as little as a few minutes, especially if this is not your first baby), or pushing can take many hours. The baby often makes very incremental movements as it navigates the pelvis, and this can take time and effort, especially the first time.

Many of my clients have been warned about "the ring of fire"—when the baby is crowning and the stretching of the vagina and perineum is especially intense. People often express concern about this along with their related concerns about vaginal tearing and stitches following their birth. During labor with my first son, as I was beginning to feel the urge to push, I had a moment where I got very afraid. I didn't want anything damaging to happen to my body, and I became overwhelmed with fear. This is not uncommon. The sensation of pushing a baby is intense. For me this felt like a moment where I threaded the needle—moving past my fear and through the intense sensation in order to meet my baby.

When you feel that big stretching, use it as a guide. In the scope of an entire pregnancy and birth, it's an incredibly small moment and it's directly followed by your baby being born. Breathe into that sensation, imagine making space, and ease your baby out. As the baby is born, some people (and some providers) enjoy having a parent-assisted delivery: if you'd like to help, or have your partner help, in the actual delivery (or "catching" of the baby), you should talk with your provider about this prenatally.

While it's common to have small tears during childbirth, perinea heal really well. I often compare the vulva and vagina to the inside of your mouth when describing to clients what to expect. When you bite your cheek it can be painful, but it also heals well and easily because the soft wet tissue inside your mouth is forgiving in this way. Similarly, your vulva and vagina are able to be stretched, and sometimes torn, and then heal without complication. Most tears during birth are called first- or second-degree tears, and they are fairly easy to heal from. Over-the-counter pain medication, taking it very easy, and not straining when you have a bowel movement (stool softeners are often suggested) are the common recommendations while these more minor tears heal.

In rare cases more serious damage happens during a vaginal birth: third- and fourth-degree tears happen in only a few percent of births, and they require more suturing and a longer amount of time to heal.[3] If you have had a third- or fourth-degree tear, I highly recommend you ask your clinical care team for detailed instructions about how to care for your healing body. My experience as a doula has been that hospitals and care providers often give far too little instructions to people with more serious tears, resulting in more pain, slower healing time, and more risk for complications. Being really vigilant about things like not straining with bowel movements (as mentioned above, stool softeners and sometimes laxatives are recommended), not lifting things or carrying anything heavy, not walking around very much in the first couple of weeks, taking pain medication and using topical numbing sprays, avoiding too much sitting and standing (favoring lying down) to decrease the pressure on your wound, cleaning your wound well with a handheld shower, and following up with your care provider, or getting a second opinion, can help enormously. Online support groups for people with more serious tears can also be helpful.

If you have a tear during birth, your epidural, if you have one, might provide sufficient numbing for stitches. If you don't have an epidural, or have pain with the epidural, your provider will use local numbing medication for pain relief. These stitches typically dissolve after a couple of weeks.

THE PLACENTA

After your baby is born, it's easy to feel a deep sense of relief that it's over, but unfortunately it's not over yet. Your baby's placenta is still inside of your uterus and needs to be birthed. For your doctor or midwife, managing the birth of the placenta and your bleeding after birth is critically important. Within thirty minutes, although often sooner, the placenta should detach from your uterine wall and come out easily, with maybe one or two pushes. It's much smaller than your baby and easy to pass.

Throughout pregnancy the placenta was attached to your uterus with blood flowing through it to your baby. When it detaches there is usually a gush of blood, and your provider or nurses might start vigorously pressing on your lower abdomen to make sure your uterus is contracting well. When the uterus contracts well, it helps slow down the bleeding and prevent a postpartum hemorrhage. A postpartum hemorrhage is a serious but rare event (studies say 1–5 percent depending on the criteria for diagnosis) in the US.[4] Your provider might use routine postpartum Pitocin, a medication typically given in a bag of IV fluids to help the uterus contract after birth and reduce the risk of a postpartum hemorrhage. You can ask ahead of time if this is routine. If the bleeding doesn't slow down, there are a wide variety of other medications and procedures that your provider can give you to slow the bleeding. If you're planning an out-of-hospital birth, asking how they manage excessive bleeding postpartum is a great question since only some midwives carry medications. Some bleeding is normal after childbirth, so expect to bleed and need pads for weeks while you heal.

If the placenta doesn't come on its own within about thirty minutes of birth, your provider might become more concerned. This is called a retained placenta, and it can be dangerous. Sometimes, the placenta has not released from the uterine wall but can be manually removed. In other cases, the placenta has detached but your cervix has begun to close a bit too soon and has "trapped" the placenta, requiring intervention to open the cervix and remove the placenta.

The most concerning form of retained placenta is a placenta accreta, where the placenta has grown too deeply into the uterine wall and becomes inseparable. A hysterectomy (removal of your uterus), and often blood transfusions, might be needed to resolve this. A previous Cesarean birth or other uterine surgery can increase the chances of a placenta accreta, although it can happen to people who've never had a uterine surgery for reasons we don't totally understand. Rising Cesarean birthrates are linked to the rise in cases of placenta accreta—in the 1950s the rate was about 1 in 30,000, but it is now closer to 1 in 700 with the greatest risk among people who've had multiple Cesarean births.[5]

Once you have birthed the placenta, you may have no further interest in it (as one client said, "Once it is no longer attached to me, I am no longer attached to it"). In most birth locations, the medical staff will dispose of your placenta for you. If you would like to see your placenta before it is discarded (or occasionally sent to pathology to be studied), you can ask your doula, nurse, or care provider to show you the placenta and explain how it works. I find that seeing your placenta can sometimes be a nice reminder of why you should slow down and give yourself several weeks of minimal activity after you give birth. It is a big organ, and it leaves a big wound inside your uterus that needs time to heal! Some people opt not to dispose of a placenta in medical waste and instead choose to bury it, often in a special place or with a special plant.

Some people opt to consume their placenta, a practice called placentophagy. Placenta consumption typically takes the form of consuming encapsulated placenta pills prepared by a hired placenta prep specialist. You can also DIY placenta pills with tutorials from the internet, cook your placenta into a stew or stir-fry, or have it made into a tincture. Some people also consume their placenta raw, often blended into a smoothie or making pill-sized pieces to swallow with water. Many believe that consuming the placenta can help prevent postpartum depression, increase milk supply, help the uterus return to pre-pregnancy size, and replenish iron lost during birth. There's little to no data about these claims or the experience of people who've consumed their placenta, so this is not currently an evidence-based practice. There's also concern about possible risks associated with placenta consumption, including risk of infection. If you're interested in placentophagy, you should ask your provider and a placenta specialist about it.

If you are interested in taking your placenta home with you from a hospital or birth center for any reason, check if your birth location restricts your access to your placenta in any way. Policies can vary hugely, and knowing this in advance can avoid any upset in the days after birth.

THE FIRST HOUR WITH YOUR BABY POSTPARTUM

After your baby is born, they can usually come directly onto your chest to be skin to skin with you. The benefits of being skin to skin are enormous and well documented. Newborns are wet at birth and can easily become cold, but being skin to skin can keep them at an optimal temperature. Babies also sync their heart rate and breathing to you when they're on your chest, two important things since breathing is a brand-new skill for them. There's much documentation about the bonding benefits of having your baby skin to skin after birth and our hormonal responses to this contact.[6] Babies get beneficial bacteria from contact with the skin after birth, bacteria that helps to colonize their immature gut.[7] Additionally, if you're chest/breastfeeding, early skin-to-skin contact helps babies nurse sooner and for longer, which can benefit your milk supply and help ensure your baby gets enough of the early milk, colostrum, to help them thrive. Some people have worried that they have missed a critical moment if immediate skin-to-skin contact is not possible (due to a Cesarean or a baby who required immediate medical attention, for example). If this is the case for you, do not worry that you have lost something you cannot get back; instead, aim to get your baby on your chest as soon as possible and you will both reap the benefits of this whenever you can.

Unless there is need for immediate medical assistance, the evidence suggests that allowing the baby's umbilical cord to remain unclamped while they lie on your chest is ideal.[8] This allows the cord blood to return to the baby before the cord is clamped and cut. When the cord is left intact, your baby's blood volume will be increased, and their iron storages are higher, which is important for healthy brain development. Delayed cord clamping also gives your baby an

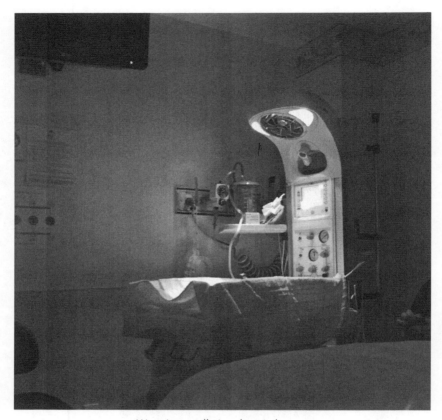

Warming cradle in a hospital room.

infusion of beneficial stem cells. If you'd like to bank your baby's cord blood in order to preserve those stem cells for possible future medical use, then more immediate cord clamping is usually recommended to collect a sufficient sample for banking. Talk to your provider about your plans and make sure they're able to support you in either delayed cord clamping or in cord blood banking, whatever you prefer.

All babies are assessed at one minute and five minutes old to quickly summarize their health on a ten-point scale for: skin color, pulse rate, reflex response to stimulation, activity, and respiratory effort. If you baby has a low Apgar score (named for Dr. Virginia Apgar) at birth, then a nurse, birth assistant, midwife, or doctor might need to further stimulate the baby, suction excess fluids, and help the baby transition to using their lungs. Some of this might be done with your baby skin to skin, or your baby might be moved to a warming cradle. If further help is needed, your baby might also be transferred to a NICU or a special nursery until the additional support is no longer needed.

The staff at the hospital often have newborn procedures they are required to perform in the first hours of your baby's life, but many of these can be done while the baby is on your chest (or being held by another person). Most hospitals take footprints, for example, which can easily be done while you hold your baby. Weighing and measuring your baby will need to be done off of your chest but can usually wait until your baby is a couple of hours old if you'd prefer. You should ask your provider about what is required at your birth location because it can vary greatly state to state and between birth locations (see "Understanding common newborn procedures" following the conclusion of this book).

CONCLUSION

Years ago, a client of mine who had studied yoga extensively wrote to me in anticipation of her birth about the rhythm of her yoga practice and the repetitive return to a resting posture. This resting posture, she told me, was the most important and advanced of all the postures, even while being seemingly the simplest. All the benefits for the mind and body are reaped in that space of relaxation, she said. She shared her sense that, similarly, in the space between contractions, she wanted to return to a meditative place to help labor progress. She also shared a mantra she'd been given by a teacher years earlier that resonated with her—*struggle less*. She'd applied that to countless moments in her life and wanted my help applying it to birth.

This concept of struggling less has been enormously helpful to me as a doula. When labor feels challenging, mentally or physically, and we struggle with it, it tends to be harder to handle. When we find a place to struggle less—to relax into it, to breathe through it—then it becomes more manageable. Labor is a time when, unlike other moments in our life, feeling physical pain isn't a sign that something is wrong. Rather, this pain has a purpose, and remembering that can be incredibly useful. Even with an epidural you might feel some pain or discomfort, or you might feel yourself struggling emotionally or physically. Coming back to a space where you struggle less can help you continue to feel more in control and more capable of coping. Part of what I like so much about this phrase is the lack of perfection in it. It's not a command to stop struggling entirely, but just to see if there are places where you can let something go, relax a little more, quiet your mind a bit, shift your mood, and struggle less.

While labor is often discussed as stages—early labor, active labor, transition, pushing—I don't find that it is usually *experienced* in stages. Stages are used by birth workers to describe birth, but they were never significant in my own births, and you might not experience them as significant either. More likely, you'll feel labor as a continuous experience of contractions becoming more frequent, stronger, and longer over time with many of the above discussed signs and sensations happening throughout the process. Whatever you feel and whatever your labor is like, expect that you might be thrilled, relieved, overwhelmed, exhausted, sore, and in love.

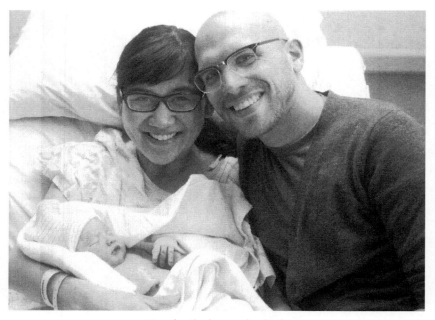

New family, hours after birth.

PACKING YOUR BAG

If you're birthing in a hospital or birth center, having your bag ready from about thirty-seven weeks on is a good idea. However, there will be things you can't put into your bag ahead of time. For these things, make a note and leave it with the bag so it's easy to add them later. The hospital or birth center should have pads, disposable underwear, and diapers, and they likely stock formula if needed.

IMPORTANT

- Any paperwork or medical records you were told to bring, your driver's license or ID, a birth plan if you have one, your insurance card, your marriage certificate (especially if you're married and have different last names or are a same-sex couple), your health care proxy (especially for unmarried or single parents), and any other legal materials as needed (such as domestic partnership or adoption paperwork)
- Toiletries (toothbrush, toothpaste, lip balm, hair ties, shampoo/conditioner, lotion, saline or contact solution, etc.) for you and your partner, and any medications you/your partner take (Tums, headache medications, prescription medications)
- Clear fluids (waters, coconut water, juice boxes, seltzer, electrolyte drinks) and, if your partner might need middle-of-the-night energy, a coffee drink, energy drink, or soda

- Nonperishable food (granola bars, protein bars, crackers, nuts, cookies, dried fruit) and also some perishables at the last minute (fruit, cheese, hard-boiled eggs) if you'd like. Remember the food is for both you and your partner in labor and afterward.
- Clothing for you postpartum (shirts that you can nurse in if you are chest/breastfeeding, shirts with yoga pants/pajama pants/leggings, nightgowns, or simple dresses). Also, your partner might want an extra outfit and a hoodie or sweater.
- Your electronics (phones, cameras, music/speakers, laptop, tablet e-reader, etc. and any cords, cables, batteries, or chargers for them). A short extension cord is often nice because the outlets are frequently in inconvenient places and an extension cord can make it possible for you to have your phone near you in bed while charging.

OPTIONAL

- Anything you want for comfort (massage oil, aromatherapy, heating pad or hot water bottle, electric candles, a picture or image, music, yoga ball, peanut ball, washcloths, a fan, straws, etc.). If you have a doula, ask what they will be bringing as they may already have some of these things for you. Your birth location may also stock some items.
- A towel (they'll typically have many towels, but you can bring your own if you want to have a nicer one for after showers or baths). To keep from having your towel confused with those provided by the birth center or hospital, I recommend any color besides white.
- A blanket (they'll typically have some for you but often a warmer/cozier one is nice). Nothing too special as it could get stained. Fleece is popular and easy to wash.
- Clothing to labor in (if you don't want to wear a hospital gown). This could be a tank top and skirt, a sleeveless nightgown, a gown ordered online specifically for birth, or something else. It should be something you don't mind throwing away.
- One or two pillows (in pillowcases that are not white) if you'd like. They'll usually have at least one for you, but more can be

nice for both labor and chest/breastfeeding. Plus, your own pillow might be more comfortable to sleep on.

- Flip-flops or disposable slippers (they'll often provide you with nonslip socks)
- Some extra bags can be useful if your birth location does not routinely provide them. These can be used to store the clothes/shoes you came in wearing, coats and winter gear if you have them, your dirty laundry from your stay, and all the items you might be sent home with (such as pads, diapers, ice packs, baby blankets, disposable underwear, etc.).
- If you are planning to keep your placenta, you'll want two- or three-gallon-sized ziplock bags and a soft cooler bag to pack the placenta into for transport.
- If you'd like to bring a gift for the nurses or your provider, which is not necessary but might be appreciated, I recommend you consider options other than cookies and chocolates (which are common). I've seen a lot of nurses very thankful for gifted pens and lip balm, for example.

FOR BABY AND GOING HOME

- A car seat that is age/weight appropriate for your baby
- They'll likely provide newborn shirts, hats, diapers, and blankets but you can also bring your own. You'll need to bring one outfit for the baby to travel home in (seasonally appropriate). This should have legs so your baby can be safely secured in a car seat.
- An outfit for you to travel home in. Remember you will still have a large belly after giving birth. Something with a very loose waist is ideal in the event you have a Cesarean birth, as anything tight on your waist will be more uncomfortable.

9

COMMON INTERVENTIONS DURING LABOR AND CHILDBIRTH

For many people, myself included, pregnancy was a vulnerable time. Preparing for labor and being in a hospital filled with doctors, machines, and medicines was intimidating. I knew I wanted to do everything I could to protect my baby and have him arrive safely, but I also wanted to do everything I could to protect myself. I didn't want those to feel like competing interests, and I didn't want the fear of something bad happening to my baby to be used as a bargaining chip to make me agree to treatments I didn't need or want.

When I was pregnant, other people often told me their birth stories, and they largely didn't help me feel more confident or comfortable. So often their stories included elements I didn't understand or want. While the childbirth class I took was helpful in preparing us for birthing in a hospital, our teacher's strong emphasis on the word "intervention" was noteworthy. She'd offer caveats about the possibility we might actually need one of these interventions, but the framing was clear: interventions were things doctors do too often and without good reason. Our work was to avoid interventions whenever possible.

These interventions, we were told, could be the beginning of a troubling "cascade of interventions"—where agreeing to one intervention leads to a domino effect of interventions, often resulting in a Cesarean birth that could have been avoided. I was nervous about the speed with which I might be asked to make decisions and my minimal understanding of the difference between a useful intervention and an unnecessary one. I was fearful I'd be overtreated.

While I trusted my providers and believed they'd only intervene if they felt it absolutely necessary, I didn't trust the hospital and the various unknown staff I'd be interacting with. My mistrust was not misplaced. There are situations where one intervention, necessary or unnecessary, then requires another (and another), and sometimes this results in an unwanted Cesarean birth. There are also other situations where an intervention helps someone avoid a Cesarean birth. And, of course, sometimes interventions, including Cesareans, save lives.

I was taught that interventions were not a positive or even neutral thing—interventions were clearly negative, an interference in the natural process. I find, as a doula, that many of my clients also have this perspective after reading childbirth books or taking classes. In this chapter, I want to bring some balance into considering interventions.

The definition of an intervention is an action taken to *improve* a situation. When used well, interventions improve health, reduce risks, and increase safety. Sometimes more medications, monitoring, and interventions are exactly what's needed. That said, as in much of life, more is not always better. There is considerable data that suggests pregnant people are overtreated and interventions are overused.[1] Not only does this not make birth safer, it makes it very difficult for you, as a patient, to feel confident that you're getting everything you need, but nothing more. Working with a provider you trust will make an enormous difference in this regard. Understanding what might be done and why can also help you participate in thoughtful conversations with your provider about your choices and what you consent to (or refuse).

In this chapter, I walk through all the routine (and some less routine) interventions in birth (in all locations) to help you understand what they're doing, why they're doing it, what the evidence tells us about how useful it is, and what risks there might be. For many of us, the routine medical procedures and practices during birth are foreign, intimidating, or concerning. In what follows, I detail both what you can expect in terms of monitoring, medications, and procedures, and the risks and benefits of each intervention so you can approach your birth with more information and, ideally, more confidence in your decision-making.

For some people, reading about these interventions will be incredibly helpful. It can be part of gaining a sense of control in childbirth and making informed choices—this is my intention and hope. That said, I want to acknowledge that, for other people, reading what follows might cause anxiety or a sense of being out of control. Recently I worked with someone who took a childbirth class she really enjoyed until the teacher showed a video of labor. The video was intended to help students visualize themselves in labor and understand the range of ways people cope with labor. It made my client feel nauseous and panicked, overwhelmed by the vulnerability of the people in the video and her own sense of how out of control she might feel in labor. She called me from the bathroom she'd retreated to partway through the video, and we talked through what she was feeling. I reminded her, as I want to remind you, that you only need to gather the information that is useful and helpful for *you*. Advocating for yourself in pregnancy and birth can also mean choosing not to watch a movie or read parts of a book.

MONITORING YOU IN PREGNANCY AND LABOR

All birth locations and providers should monitor your basic indexes of health. It's typical for both midwives and doctors to check your blood pressure during prenatal visits and periodically during labor. Additionally, it's common to monitor your temperature during labor and often also your pulse and the oxygen levels in your blood. Checking your urine and blood is also common during pregnancy and in labor, and toward the end of pregnancy you'll also be checked for something called group beta strep (GBS). During pregnancy and labor, there will be increased activity to manage your baby's well-being. Below, I detail the ways you'll likely be monitored and checked to help you understand what to expect, why they're doing it, and what the results of the tests might mean.

BLOOD TESTS IN PREGNANCY AND LABOR

Midwives and doctors, supporting birth in every location, routinely take blood early in pregnancy to test for a wide variety of things. They check your complete blood count, which can help identify anemia (low iron), your white blood cell count to help identify if your body is fighting disease or infection, and your platelet count (for blood clotting). Additionally, they check your blood type and your Rh factor (a protein in your red blood cells), and potentially screen for possible genetic disorders you might be a carrier for (if this wasn't done prior to pregnancy). This information can help tailor recommendations, such as suggesting iron supplementation if you're anemic, and it can help guide clinical treatment, such as offering Rhogam if you're Rh negative (to prevent the possibility of your immune system reacting to the baby's Rh-positive blood).

Blood tests can also be used to check your immunity to things like rubella (German measles) and infections such as hepatitis, HIV, Zika, or syphilis. Blood tests in early pregnancy are also used to check for your fetus's sex; abnormalities of the sex chromosomes (such as Klinefelter and Turner syndromes); trisomy 21 (Down syndrome), 18, and 13; and other common and rare chromosomal abnormalities. These tests are not 100 percent accurate, and getting a positive result is usually followed by genetic counseling and often more invasive tests like chorionic villus sampling (CVS) or amniocentesis. CVS and amniocentesis involve drawing samples of the placenta (CVS) or the amniotic fluid (amniocentesis) to check for chromosomal abnormalities and genetic disorders, and with amniocentesis neural tube defects can also be checked. Speak with your provider about your risks, whether these tests are recommended for you, and about accessing a genetic counselor if you'd like help making decisions.

Later in pregnancy, blood tests are routinely given between twenty-four and twenty-eight weeks to check the amount of glucose in your blood and screen for gestational diabetes (affecting about 6 percent of pregnant people in the US).[2] Often the first test to screen for gestational diabetes involves consuming a very sweet drink, waiting an hour, and then having your blood drawn. This test is not used to diagnose gestational diabetes but rather to screen for people who should have follow up testing—the glucose tolerance test (GTT). This test involves eight hours of fasting, having a fasting blood test, consuming the sweet drink again, and having your blood drawn three times over the next three hours. Too high of a glucose reading on any two of these four blood tests is the criteria for diagnosing gestational diabetes.

In labor and prior to Cesarean births, hospitals routinely draw more blood to check your complete blood count and blood type again, plus screen for infection (and potentially drugs in your system). This blood is typically drawn either the day before a planned Cesarean birth or upon admission to the hospital in labor or for an induction. Some birth centers, especially those inside hospitals, routinely draw blood in labor. Freestanding birth centers and homebirth midwives rarely draw blood in labor. Postpartum blood draws might also be recommended, especially if you lost more blood than expected during your birth and your provider is concerned.

BLOOD PRESSURE MONITORING

In all birth locations and with all types of providers, it's standard to monitor your blood pressure both in pregnancy and in labor, as high blood pressure can cause concerns for both you and your baby. A cuff will be wrapped around your upper arm and inflated, often squeezing your arm very tightly. There are two numbers recorded in a blood pressure reading: the systolic (the top, larger number) and the diastolic (the bottom, smaller number). The systolic number measures the force of your heart pushing blood through your arteries and the pressure this creates on your blood vessels. The diastolic reading is the pressure on the arteries when the heart rests between beats.

Your care provider will want to confirm that your blood pressure is normal, as elevated blood pressure in pregnancy and in labor can indicate more serious health concerns. Similarly, very low blood pressure can be concerning and is a common side effect of epidurals. Because of this, frequent blood pressure readings typically accompany epidurals.

Sometimes people will have a false high blood pressure reading because they're anxious, in pain, or moving too much during the reading. My client Kay, for example, found that her blood pressure reading was high at every OB appointment if they took her pressure when she first arrived. The appointments made her anxious, but she became more relaxed after seeing the doctor and hearing that everything was going well. If your first reading is high, like Kay's, retesting to confirm that the high reading is accurate is standard. If you believe you might be testing high because you're nervous or anxious, it can be good to ask for a few minutes to lie down and slow your breathing before retesting. With Kay, she requested they take her blood pressure reading at the end of visits, rather than the beginning, and all her readings were normal after that. Additionally, sometimes the monitor itself isn't working well or is not sized well for your arm, so it is good to make sure the person checking your blood pressure (often a nurse) is using a well-sized cuff and feels confident the reading is accurate.

You should expect to have your blood pressure checked periodically throughout labor. How often it's done will depend on your provider and birth location, whether your numbers are in the normal range, and if you've gotten epidural pain medication or a spinal block for a Cesarean birth. You might have one or two blood pressure readings total in labor, or you might have blood pressure readings multiple times per hour. You should expect that blood pressure readings will continue after you give birth. This is especially true in the hospital where it's common to read the blood pressure several times per hour in the first hours after birth and periodically throughout your entire stay.

TEMPERATURE

Your midwife, a nurse, or a medical assistant will take your temperature periodically throughout labor either under your tongue, under your armpit, or sometimes with a special sensor swiped across your forehead. If you have a catheter in your bladder for any reason, some hospitals monitor your temperature through the catheter. Different care providers and birth locations monitor temperature with different frequency—sometimes they check it once, other times you might have it checked hourly or more. Usually temperature checks are more frequent once your water has broken and especially if it has been broken for a long time. Monitoring your temperature is a great way to watch for signs of infection and dehydration.

PULSE AND OXYGEN SATURATION

Some providers monitor your pulse during labor by simply counting with their fingers on your wrist or neck. In hospitals, and some birth centers, it's common to have a pulse oximeter read both your pulse and oxygen saturation levels. This reading is done with a sensor on your finger.

Monitoring your pulse during labor (and postpartum) can be helpful for a variety of reasons including checking for signs of dehydration, fever, and blood loss, all of which can increase your pulse. It can also help ensure the accuracy of external fetal monitors. These monitors can accidentally pick up your heart rate instead of your baby's heart rate, causing unnecessary concern. Your baby's heart rate should be higher than yours, and a misreading can suggest your baby is distressed when they're fine. This isn't uncommon. Monitoring your pulse can help providers to distinguish between a low fetal heart rate and monitors that are accidentally picking up your heart rate.

URINALYSIS

During pregnancy you will be asked—likely many times, especially if you are seeing an OB—to pee in a cup so your provider can analyze your urine. There's lots of useful information that can be accessed through urine, such as signs of dehydration, diabetes, bacteria, disease, and infections like sexually transmitted infections and urinary tract infections. Sometimes your urine is also tested for signs of recreational drug use depending on your provider and birth location.

GROUP BETA STREP SWAB

Occasionally providers will notice that you have a bacterium called group beta strep (GBS) present in your urine during the routine urinalysis discussed above. More commonly, your provider will use an extralong Q-tip-like swab on your vagina and rectum to see if you have what is called a colonization of GBS. This is typically done late in pregnancy, around thirty-six weeks. While having a colonization of this bacteria is a type of infection, it's not related to infections you might be more aware of or bothered by, such as sexually transmitted infections, yeast infections, or urinary tract infections. And although they share a name, strep throat and group beta strep aren't the same thing. If you're colonized with GBS, you'll likely have no symptoms. Most people only become aware of GBS because they're tested in pregnancy, and about 25 percent of pregnant people test positive for it.[3]

While being colonized with GBS is not problematic for you, it can be serious for your baby. GBS infection can cause complications in babies such as sepsis, pneumonia, meningitis, breathing problems, and more. Even if you're colonized, thankfully your baby will likely not get GBS. For people who test positive and are *not* treated for it, about 1 in 200 babies will get GBS. If you have antibiotic treatment for the GBS, this rate is even lower with only about 1 in every 4,000 babies getting GBS.[4]

Given the big difference in risk for the baby when pregnant people are not treated for GBS, the clinical recommendation is usually to get IV antibiotics during your labor. Antibiotic treatment is most effective when it is started after your water breaks or at least four hours before you give birth so you can get two doses of antibiotics, given four hours apart.[5] IV antibiotics are available in hospitals and also out of hospital if your midwife is a CNM, but they're often not available if you are working with other types of midwives.

Many people are unhappy about IV antibiotics—both because it requires having an IV and because they're concerned about the risks of antibiotic treatment for themselves and for their baby. In my experience, the antibiotics take about thirty minutes to get, and the IV doesn't need to be attached after that. As for concerns about antibiotic treatment, there is data to suggest that IV antibiotics do temporarily reduce the beneficial bacteria in a newborn's gut (although it seems to recover within a few months).[6] These effects are lessened by having your baby skin to skin and nursing. And this data is very new: our sense of what the impact is could change greatly with new data.

Minimizing the number of antibiotic doses you receive might be possible if you are concerned about antibiotics in your labor. The data is clear: two doses four hours apart is far more effective than one dose, but beyond that, you may not need more.[7] Talk to your provider about timing the beginning of antibiotic treatment to reduce the doses you receive.

Another concern is the possibility you don't have GBS and antibiotics are unnecessary. This is possible—studies suggest about 16 percent of people treated with antibiotics for GBS in labor actually no longer had GBS, even though the initial test was positive.[8] Similarly, it's possible (although much less probable) to test negative for GBS but develop a colonization by the time you give birth. Some providers will retest depending on the amount of time since your last test—speak with your provider if you'd like to be retested for any reason.

You can refuse treatment with antibiotics after testing positive for GBS—you don't have to consent to any treatment you don't want. If this is something you're considering, it can be helpful to know that some people are at an even higher risk for having a baby with GBS. Risk factors that increase the possibility your baby will get GBS from you include having GBS in your urine during pregnancy, your water breaking before thirty-seven weeks, having your water broken for more than eighteen hours before giving birth, a fever during labor, and having one baby with GBS already.[9] If you've refused treatment with antibiotics and you become higher risk during your labor, such as developing a fever or having your water broken for longer than eighteen hours, then accepting antibiotic treatment is even more strongly advised.

If your provider doesn't test for GBS or offer treatment and you're concerned, ask if testing is available or consider switching to a provider who will test and treat.

IV ACCESS AND IV FLUIDS

In hospitals, it's routine to want all laboring patients to have a catheter inserted into a vein on your forearm or hand and secured with tape to hold it in place. This is variously called a hep lock, a saline lock, or a med lock, among other names, but they all refer to the same thing—IV access in the event that you need fluids, medications, or in rare cases, a blood transfusion. In birth centers and at home, IV access is uncommon unless you have GBS.

Sometimes continuous IV fluids are required, not just the IV access. Typically the IV fluid you will be given is called a lactated ringer (or LR), which is a mixture of water with sodium chloride, sodium lactate, potassium chloride, and calcium chloride. LRs are usually given to people who need electrolytes or who have low blood pressure, and are routinely used in labor for both of these reasons.

If you've been throwing up throughout labor, IV fluids might be helpful and can sometimes give you more energy to continue laboring. Anya, for example, had planned to refuse IV fluids in favor of staying hydrated by drinking, but in labor she found that drinking more than a sip of fluid caused her to throw up.

The combination of so much vomiting and becoming dehydrated made her feel miserable and weak. She said, "I reluctantly agreed to a bag of IV fluids—an intervention I'd imagined really wanting to avoid—and in 20 minutes I was already feeling more able to handle my contractions and less exhausted and depleted. It really helped me continue to labor and I'm really grateful for it."

If you have an epidural for labor or anesthesia for a Cesarean birth, continuous IV fluids will usually be required. If your baby appears to be sleepy or distressed on the monitors, you will often be given IV fluids to see if this helps. IV fluids are also common postpartum in many hospitals. Some people find that they are given so many bags of IV fluids during the course of labor and postpartum that they become very swollen in the days after giving birth. Speak to your provider about what is standard in your birth location, what your provider recommends, and any concerns you have about IV access or IV fluids.

MONITORING THE BABY

In all birth locations, with all providers, a certain amount of monitoring of the baby should be expected both prenatally and in labor. Your provider will want to listen to the fetal heartbeat during pregnancy to verify that the baby is doing well and not exhibiting signs of distress. Similarly, in labor, monitoring of the baby's heartbeat is standard. How much, and in what form, will depend on the birth location and your provider—with homebirths and birth centers requiring the least monitoring and hospitals requiring the most.

There are several ways to monitor your baby: a handheld Doppler or a Pinard horn, an external electronic fetal monitor (EFM), or an internal fetal monitor. During labor, most providers use one of these methods to track the baby's heartbeat. This is combined with some form of contraction monitoring. Your provider may observe your contraction while monitoring the baby (very common in out-of-hospital births and with midwives), or they might use either an external monitor (called a toco) or an internal contraction monitor. Monitoring the baby's reaction to contractions lets your provider see how your baby is tolerating labor. Below, I describe these monitoring methods along with the pros and cons of each.

External Auscultation: Pinard Horn or Handheld Doppler

If a provider has ever used a stethoscope on you during a routine exam, you already know what auscultation is, even if the word is not familiar. Auscultation is listening to sounds from inside your body—your heart, lungs, or other organs—as part of medical treatment. Some providers use a tool similar to a stethoscope, called a Pinard horn (or sometimes called a fetoscope, although that term is also used for a surgical treatment, so it can be confusing), to listen to the heartbeat of your developing baby. It has about an eight-inch-long "horn" that looks like a tiny trumpet and is placed on your belly to amplify sound. It was invented by a French obstetrician in the nineteenth century, but these days I've only seen midwives using this tool (and rarely). Some find it uncomfortable because it needs to be pressed firmly into the belly to hear the heartbeat.

More commonly, care providers use a small, portable handheld monitor to listen to the heartbeat. These monitors rely on Doppler ultrasound, using sound waves to detect and communicate movements inside your body—in this case the movement of your baby's heart as it beats. This monitor translates these movements into an audible sound so you and your provider can both hear the heartbeat. The shared experience of hearing the heartbeat is often something people cite as an advantage of these handheld Doppler monitors over the Pinard horn, where only one person can hear the heartbeat (at a time). Handheld Dopplers also usually have a digital display of the beats per minute for your provider to read.

Handheld Dopplers are popular among providers who see patients in their homes, such as homebirth midwives, and for use in-office visits. Because hand-

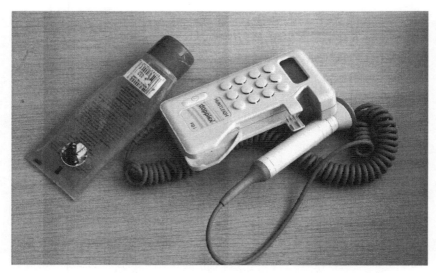

A handheld Doppler with aloe gel used by a homebirth midwife.

held Dopplers can be waterproof, providers can use them to monitor people laboring in birth tubs. If you are moving around a lot in labor, a handheld Doppler can help your provider go wherever you are, rather than needing you to come to them. Some hospitals stock them for nurses to use when a patient is in the shower or moving around to cope with labor, but many hospitals do not.

Handheld Dopplers are not practical when continuous monitoring is required. They're also more difficult to use if your provider needs to perform other tasks at the same time. There are concerns about parents buying these handheld devices for personal use to listen to their baby between appointments. Use without training can result in misinterpreting what you're hearing—causing concern when there's no reason for alarm, and also potentially offering false reassurance when there might be cause for concern.

External Electronic Fetal Monitoring and Toco

The most common form of fetal monitoring in the US is two disc-shaped monitors placed on your belly and held in place with either straps or a band. This might be done during pregnancy (called a nonstress test), and it's routinely done in labor. One monitor is for the baby's heart rate and uses Doppler ultrasound, like the handheld monitor described above. The second monitor is a simple pressure sensor called a toco (short for tocodynamometer or tocometer) placed on your belly to help detect when your uterus contracts (but it also records anything else that changes pressure like a cough, sitting up, laughing, throwing up, etc.). The toco, when working well, records when contractions happen and how long they last (frequency and duration) but cannot measure the intensity or strength of contractions.

Both monitors will need to be adjusted repeatedly throughout labor because they rely on being placed well to function. If the baby moves, for example, the heart monitor might need to be moved to pick up the baby's heartbeat. Similarly, if the toco is not able to sense the change in your uterus when you contract, it will chart that there are no contractions. Further, they don't work equally well on all bodies and can create a false sense of danger, resulting in unnecessary concern and intervention.

Frances, for example, described herself as a plus-sized woman and said she was minutes away from having an unnecessary Cesarean because her nurse could no longer hear her baby's heartbeat when the baby moved lower. Unable to hear the baby's heartbeat, her nurse panicked and called in her doctors. The doctors told the staff to prepare an operating room for immediate delivery. Frances recalled her doula taking the monitor in this chaos and shoving it at an angle into the bottom of her belly right above her pelvic bones. A booming sound (the volume was turned up during the frantic search for the baby's heartbeat) filled the room. "My baby's totally normal heartbeat calmed everyone down and canceled the emergency Cesarean." Frances's experience can happen to anyone—regardless of size—although it's more common for larger people because the monitors don't work as well on our bodies.[10] Being aware of this can help you advocate for yourself if you find that your providers are becoming nervous about your baby.

Both monitors are attached by cables that are connected to a station next to the hospital bed that usually has a computer, computer screen (or several), and a printer where the "tracing" is recorded and visible for the medical staff (and you) to view. Collectively, this monitoring unit is called a cardiotocograph, although I never hear this term used in hospitals. Everyone seems to prefer calling them "the monitors." There are wireless versions of these monitors available in some hospitals, which can allow you greater mobility while still being monitored.

In hospitals, it's common for everyone to be monitored for at least twenty to thirty minutes upon arriving and periodically throughout labor. This is called intermittent monitoring, and it's a safe and effective way to monitor low-risk patients laboring without pain medication or labor-inducing medicines. If these monitors are placed on you and remain on you throughout your entire labor, this is continuous monitoring. Continuous monitoring is considered a better option if there's concern for how the baby is tolerating labor, if you're higher risk (attempting a VBAC, for example), are receiving pain medication, or you're being induced.

Some providers and birth locations never allow intermittent monitoring, continuously monitoring all patients regardless of risk or indication. This is not an evidence-based practice. Routine continuous fetal monitoring doesn't improve outcomes for you or your baby.[11] If you'd like intermittent monitoring, make sure your birth location and provider commonly use intermittent monitoring.

Internal Fetal Monitoring and the Intrauterine Pressure Catheter

Each of the external monitors that are part of the cardiotocograph—the fetal monitor and the toco—can be swapped for an internal version if more (or better) information is needed. If the fetal monitor isn't picking up the baby's heart rate accurately, your provider might place an internal fetal monitor directly on your baby. This monitor has a thin spiral of metal wire on one end that your provider

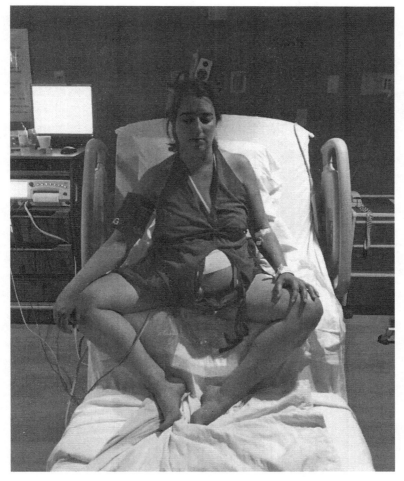

Laboring with fetal monitors, blood pressure cuff, and hep lock.

will guide into place on top of your baby's skull with their fingers. Once they've gotten the monitor in contact with the top of the head, they rotate or screw the thin metal wire into your baby's scalp. I know this sounds pretty awful, and I've never explained it to anyone without an immediate negative reaction, but it is a very tiny piece of metal that leaves a pinprick-sized spot on your baby's head, and it's typically removed as they're being born. It's an electronic transducer, or electrode, that's able to send a direct signal, very accurately recording the heartbeat. Unlike external Doppler monitors, the shape of the pregnant person's body and your movement won't impact accuracy. You'll have a thin tube coming out of your vagina and taped to your leg, which can be annoying, but it should not be painful or limiting in any way.

Similarly, if the external toco monitor isn't able to accurately record the frequency of contractions, or if there's a question about the strength of the contraction, an internal monitor might be used. An intrauterine pressure catheter (IUPC) is a thin plastic tube that your provider can thread into your cervix, past your baby's head, and into the amniotic space. It has a pressure transducer on the tip that can measure the strength of contractions, as well as the frequency and duration. Like the internal fetal monitor, having an IUPC will mean there's a thin tube coming out of your vagina and taped to your leg. It also shouldn't be painful or limiting in any way.

While there's no reason to use an IUPC in the vast majority of labors, and it doesn't improve outcomes to use it routinely, there are situations where it's a great tool. For example, if your contractions are frequent but very weak, an IUPC can help your provider use Pitocin to increase the strength of your contractions rather than having a Cesarean birth for "failure to progress." This use of it can increase the chances of a vaginal birth.

In order to use either of these monitors your water must be broken, so converting from an external monitor to an internal one sometimes requires your care provider to break your water. On the whole, external fetal monitors are generally preferred because they're less invasive and carry fewer risks (anything placed inside your cervix increases the risk of infection).

MEDICAL PAIN RELIEF

If you'd like medical pain relief, there are many options—although what's available to you might depend on your birth location and your health history. Speak with your provider prenatally about what options will be available, any restrictions specific to your health, and any recommendations they have for which medical pain relief options might be best. Below, I describe the most common medical pain relief options used in hospitals (and sometimes birth centers) and some of the pros and cons, as well as risks and benefits, of each option.

Epidural

The most popular medical pain relief for labor is the epidural block (usually just called an epidural). The exact number of people who currently opt for an epidural during labor varies enormously from state to state and hospital to hospital. Rates range from as low as 20 percent to more than 90 percent. Countrywide, at least half of pregnant people opt for an epidural during labor.[12]

In my experience, many people are a bit anxious about having an epidural. They might be uncomfortable with the idea of being numb or less mobile, worried that having an epidural will increase the risk of needing other interventions, concerned it might impact their baby, nervous about the needle, and sometimes also conflicted about using pain medication at all. Ultimately the decision to have an epidural, or not, is yours to make. In what follows, I provide a straightforward, nonjudgmental, evidence-based description of epidurals and other pain relief options.

An epidural is a small catheter (a thin flexible plastic tube) that is placed in the space near your spinal cord in your lower back. In order to place the epidural, usually you sit upright on the bed and curve your back, slumping your shoulders so your lower back is pushed out toward the anesthesiologist. They'll clean your back with a cold, wet solution and place a sterile plastic drape on your back. Typically they'll inject local numbing medication into your lower back. This is usually the only part of the experience that's painful. It feels like a pinch, followed by a brief burning or stinging sensation.

After this, that area of your back should be numb, and you'll only feel pushing or pressure sensations while they find the right place to insert the needle. After the needle is inserted, they thread a small plastic catheter (the size of thin spaghetti) into the epidural space and remove the needle entirely, leaving only the catheter inside you. This catheter is used to deliver a cocktail of pain medications to provide a regional nerve block (meaning the pain signals these nerves usually send to the brain are blocked). This nerve block lessens or entirely masks the sensation of contractions, allowing you to labor with little or no pain.

The epidural is the catheter through which pain medications reach your nerves, but the medications that are delivered through the epidural vary. The medications you are given will vary depending on the hospital you give birth at—even here in NYC where hospitals can be just blocks apart, the medications vary slightly. Additionally, the medication you're given might vary because the initial medications didn't provide sufficient relief and other medications were needed to get you comfortable. Common ingredients in the epidural cocktail include a local anesthetic such as bupivacaine or lidocaine, and an opioid or narcotic such as fentanyl, sufentanil, or morphine, among others. If you'd like to know which medications you'll receive, consult your provider or ask to meet with the anesthesiologists who'll be caring for you during labor.

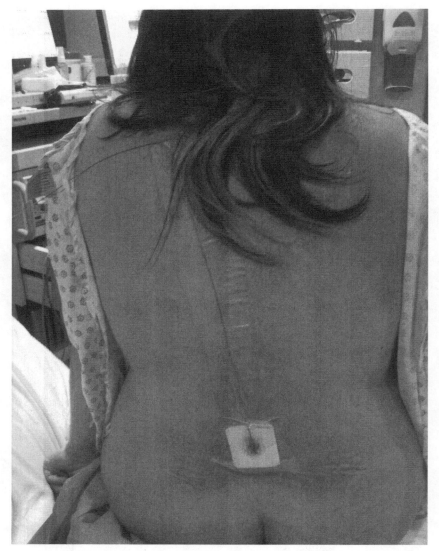

Epidural catheter placed in lower back and secured with tape.

Most hospitals place limitations on who can be with you when you're getting an epidural. Sometimes this is described as necessary for space reasons (because there are more doctors in the room), and sometimes it's described as a way to minimize the risk (because fewer people will mean fewer germs). My experience is that this varies from hospital to hospital and even within hospitals among different anesthesiologists. You might have two people with you, one person, or none of your support people. If it's important to you who'll be with you during the placement of the epidural, check with your provider and the anesthesia department at your hospital.

A nurse will always remain with you, in addition to one or two anesthesiologists. If there are two anesthesiologists in the room, it might be because you're at a teaching hospital and one is an attending doctor (a senior doctor) and one is a resident (a doctor still completing their education under supervision). If it's important to you to know who'll be placing the epidural, check with your provider or the anesthesia department at your hospital to see if residents routinely give epidurals. If you'd prefer to have the attending place it, it's always your right to request this.

One possible side effect of an epidural is a drop in blood pressure. Most hospitals require that you've already had some IV fluids before the epidural is placed, to help prevent your blood pressure from dropping too much. You'll also need to have continuous IV fluids the entire time you have the epidural, and it's common to monitor your blood pressure several times an hour throughout the rest of labor after the epidural is placed.

Most people also need a catheter to drain urine from their bladder after having an epidural. You might not feel the sensation of needing to pee and might not have the muscle control needed to urinate with an epidural. The catheter will prevent your bladder from getting too full (full bladders can slow labor and increase your risk of bleeding postpartum). Speak to your care provider about how they recommend this be managed.

Some hospitals offer what is called a "walking epidural," but don't be fooled by this language—in the vast majority of cases this doesn't mean you'll actually be able to have epidural pain medication and continue to walk. Walking epidurals are largely the same as epidurals, but the medication is administered slightly differently, so you might have more mobility in your legs and find changing positions easier. That said, in my experience, patients are usually required to stay in bed once they've had an epidural. You can ask about the policies at your birth location.

The most common side effects of an epidural include itching, soreness in the lower back where it was placed, and the risk of a specific type of headache that appears in the first day or two postpartum. The risk of a spinal headache is about 1 percent[13] (but check with your anesthesia department to confirm their rate and anything about your health that might increase or decrease your odds). Spinal headaches are most often treated with caffeine and Tylenol. If this isn't

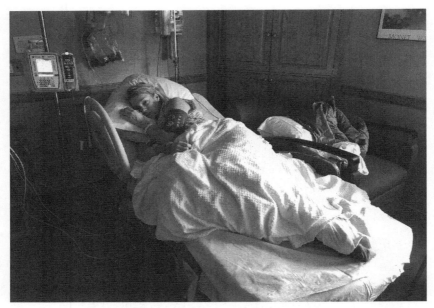

Resting with an epidural after many hours of labor.

enough, they can perform a second procedure, much like the original epidural, to create a blood patch and resolve the headache.

Many pregnant people I have spoken with worry that there's an optimal time to get an epidural, fearful that getting it too early will result in a Cesarean birth but also concerned about not getting one at all if they delay too long. Multiple studies have shown that epidurals do not significantly increase the risk of Cesareans and that timing of the epidural did not change the Cesarean birth rate or other obstetric outcomes.[14] In my experience, many care providers counsel patients that medication (Pitocin usually) might be needed if contractions space out after getting an epidural, and the use of Pitocin with epidurals is common.

Some of my clients only elect to have an epidural after laboring for many hours without. Others opt for an epidural at the first signs of labor or the beginning stages of an induction. When you would like pain relief is a very personal decision, best made by you based on what you are feeling and what you would like to be feeling.

Many people also worry that an epidural will make pushing take longer and increase their risk of assisted vaginal delivery (forceps and vacuums). Recent studies show that there is no difference in assisted vaginal deliveries with epidurals in the last decade and have similarly shown minimal (fourteen-minute to six-minute) difference in pushing time with an epidural.[15]

There are some studies that suggest babies don't nurse as well when an epidural was used in labor, but we likely do not have enough good data to fully understand the impacts, if any, of epidurals on chest/breastfeeding. Studies on chest/breastfeeding impact have often combined data on different types of pain relief options and used different methods to evaluate success or trouble, making it hard to know what the impact might be. In practice, the variables of each labor and birth and each lactating parent and newborn pair are so complex that it feels nearly impossible to isolate out one factor, such as the epidural. In my own practice, I have not seen a significant difference in chest/breastfeeding troubles or success that I feel can be attributed to having, or not having, an epidural.

Finally, it's useful to know that not every epidural is perfect, and even with an epidural you may continue to feel some discomfort or pain. Speak with your anesthesiologist about managing this if you're uncomfortable. Hospitals differ in how they manage this, including having patients administer extra doses of pain medication to themselves and doctors providing additional pain medication throughout labor when requested.

Your anesthesiologist can speak with you about rare risks—such as nerve damage, infection, bleeding—and how they reduce these risks. This should be part of the consent process before the procedure.

The benefits of an epidural are centrally about the pain relief it provides and often the rest this pain relief allows (although on more rare occasions I have also seen an epidural recommended to help reduce blood pressure in a client with high pressure readings). If labor has been long, or you're exhausted, an epidural can allow you to take a nap while labor continues. Epidurals, because they work at the nerve level, allow you to stay alert and present for labor, which many people appreciate. Your epidural can also be used for more comprehensive numbing in the event that a Cesarean birth becomes recommended or required during the course of labor. For many people, having an epidural is key to their positive experience of childbirth.

Sometimes an epidural is not available for a variety of reasons. They are not routinely available outside of hospitals. An epidural might not be available for you because of your own health issues—very low platelet counts or being on blood thinners, for example. Sometimes your anatomy or history makes it impossible for them to access the epidural space—certain back surgeries, for example. Further, some hospitals or providers might place restrictions on when an epidural is available, such as a stage of labor you must be in. If having an epidural is important to you, you may want to speak with your provider more about possible restrictions and what alternatives might be available.

Nitrous Oxide

Another option for pain relief during labor is nitrous oxide, commonly called nitrous or laughing gas. Nitrous oxide has been used during labor in the US for a long time, but it's much more commonly used in Europe. In Europe, it's often called "air and gas" or Entonox, and is a mixture of 50 percent nitrous oxide and 50 percent oxygen. In NYC, like much of the country, access to nitrous oxide in labor is uncommon but increasing in the last few years (but only at some hospitals and birth centers). That said, it's a popular form of pain relief for those who have access to it, and unlike epidurals, it's often available in birth centers (and sometimes homebirths).

Using nitrous oxide during labor usually involves placing a face mask over your nose and mouth during a contraction to breathe in a mixture of nitrous oxide and oxygen (it's safest to use only 50 percent nitrous at the most). Some people find holding the mask to their face and learning how to breathe with it confusing, but with practice it usually becomes easy. It's a fast-acting drug, providing nearly immediate partial pain relief and then wearing off quickly. The goal of nitrous oxide is not to provide complete pain relief, the way an epidural might. Nitrous oxide reduces the experience of pain without getting rid of it. For most people who use nitrous oxide during labor, it's used to provide short-term relief—perhaps for as little as ten to twenty minutes or up to a few hours. Hannah, for example, said she was "trying to go without an epidural" and used nitrous oxide for thirty minutes to get "through my transition until I was ready to push." She described it as "taking the edge off at the end" and providing "a bit of relief" to help her finish.

There are a number of documented benefits to using nitrous oxide over other forms of medical pain relief during labor, including no disruption of oxytocin production or the progress of labor, no impact on nursing, and no increased risk to the baby for needing resuscitation[16] (see below for this concern with narcotics). Additionally, because it's self-administered and fast acting, it's totally up to you how much to use and when to stop. If you don't like it you can stop, and the effects wear off in minutes. If it's not enough relief, you can switch to another pain relief option (which is not uncommon: one study showed approximately 40 percent of people who used nitrous oxide also got an epidural).[17]

While nitrous oxide is considered safe to use during labor, it's not entirely without risks. The most common side effects are sleepiness, dizziness, nausea, and vomiting. I haven't personally seen it make anyone feel sick or vomit, but I've seen it make many people a bit light headed and tired. For this reason, your provider will likely require you to sit or lie down. That said, because it wears off quickly, this requirement is typically temporary, and within minutes of using the nitrous oxide you're free to get up and move around however you'd like. There are specific conditions that making using nitrous oxide unsafe, such as vitamin B12 deficiency or recent ear surgery, among others. Speak with your provider about any limitations that might be placed because of your health.

Opiates, Opioids, and Narcotics

Opiates, opioids, and narcotics are also a common form of pain relief during labor offered to pregnant people, usually only in hospitals but occasionally elsewhere. Medications such as Stadol, fentanyl, Nubain, and Demerol are used and can be given in small doses to increase relaxation, help you rest, reduce anxiety, and make the pain of labor more manageable. These medications are sometimes used prior to getting an epidural, and other times they're used instead of an epidural. They're given either through the IV access, or they can be given as a shot in your muscle (called IM, or intramuscular).

I have attended nearly six hundred births in NYC and only seen IM or IV pain medication a handful of times, but national estimates of narcotic and opioid use in labor are 40–60 percent.[18] NYC hospitals have much higher rates of epidural use instead. When I've seen IV pain medication offered to clients, it's always been in very early labor and always as a step prior to getting an epidural, not as an alternative to an epidural. This isn't the case in much of the country where narcotics and opioids are the most common form of labor pain relief and are used almost exclusively instead of epidurals. Because IV and IM pain medications can be given by a nurse and don't require a specialist, they're most common in rural areas, smaller hospitals, and hospitals that don't have anesthesiologists dedicated exclusively to labor and delivery.

There are some advantages to using IV or IM pain medication, such as the speed they take effect and the ease of giving them. An IM shot of pain medication doesn't even require IV access and can be given quickly by any medical personnel. Depending on the medication and the dose, they also wear off relatively quickly, which can have similar advantages to the nitrous oxide described above—taking the edge off to help someone get through a short period of time in labor. These medications also don't create any numbness and don't have any impact on the ability of a laboring person to feel the urge to push.

Some of the downsides of IV and IM pain medication include nausea, vomiting, itching, dizziness, sedation, and possible breathing issues for the pregnant person. It also usually creates a feeling of being groggy, fuzzy, or high. For some people this is a welcome feeling, while others might find it unpleasant. Further, because these medications do cross the placenta, your baby also experiences the effects of these medications. This can impact your baby's nervous system, create respiratory depression, alter neurological behavior, decrease the baby's ability to regulate their body temperature, and make early chest/breastfeeding more difficult. This is much less of a concern if the medication has totally worn off before birth, but if the medication is still in your system, your baby might need medical assistance to counteract the effects. Your baby might need help with breathing and might be given a small dose of the drug naloxone, used to block the effects of opioids and quickly (within minutes) reverse respiratory depression.

Transcutaneous Electrical Nerve Stimulation (TENS) Unit

Although fairly uncommon in the US, another option for pain management in labor is a TENS unit. These are nonprescription, handheld devices often used for treating other types of pain, such as back pain. You place several pads on your back that are attached to electrical leads, connected to the TENS unit. When you begin to have a contraction, you press a button to send a small electrical pulse. This tiny pulse gives you a tingling or buzzing feeling and helps prevent pain signals from reaching your brain. This pulse can reduce the experience of pain and stimulate your body to release hormones such as endorphins. Endorphins help reduce pain and increase feelings of happiness or pleasure (your body tends to release a lot of these during a difficult workout or an orgasm, for example, and in labor you have a lot of endorphins). You can set it up to give you a low level of stimulation constantly and adjust the strength of the pulse during contractions as desired.

For many people, a TENS unit can help them feel more in control of labor, offering a nice distraction from contractions and reducing the intensity of sensation. Among my clients who've used them, I've found them more effective in early labor, when the sensations are milder. For some, they're a nice tool for managing labor prior to other pain management options and less frequently, they are used for the entire labor.

TENS units are not recommended for people with epilepsy or heart problems, and they can't be used in the water or on broken skin or a healing scar. They're not routinely provided by hospitals or birth centers, but are available

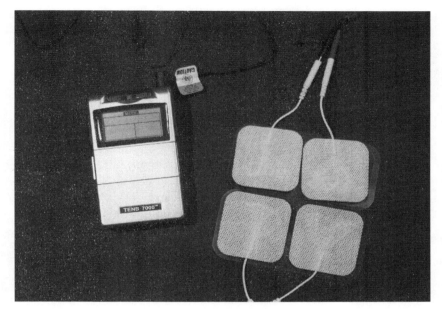

A TENS unit for pain relief in labor.

easily for purchase (and your doula or midwife might have one). Speak with your provider in advance if you'd like to use a TENS unit. A TENS unit might be new to your provider, and it's best to not surprise them with it in labor.

Sterile Water Injections (SWI)

Another less commonly used intervention is sterile water injections (SWI) into the lower back to relieve back pain during labor. Although this is almost exclusively done by midwives, any practitioner in any birth location could do it. For this procedure, four injections are made under the skin of your lower back (often two people each administer two shots simultaneously). The injections cause a brief (less than a minute) intense stinging or burning sensation, like being stung by a bee. This wears off quickly, and most people experience a lot of relief from back pain (but not other pain) for an hour or two after the SWI are placed.

This is a very simple procedure and can be repeated as many times as needed without adverse impact. There are no known side effects (beyond the small risk of infection anytime you break the skin) or reasons for concern for either you or your baby. It doesn't impact mobility or your mental state and has no impact on labor progress. This is an incredibly safe and fairly effective means of relieving back pain during labor, and it likely should be used more than it currently is. If you're interested in this option for your birth, speak with your provider ahead of time. Even if they're not already offering SWI, they could quickly learn how and potentially make it available for you.

Other Pain Relief Interventions/Options

Your birth location or birth team might also offer other forms of pain relief during labor including nonmedical support such as massage, breathing help, position changes, showers, labor tubs, yoga or birth balls, peanut balls, ice packs, and more. Additionally, some birth locations or providers might offer acupuncture—a form of traditional Chinese medicine where specific points in the body are stimulated, usually with thin needles, to help with a wide variety of things including labor progress and pain relief. Your provider might suggest over-the-counter sleep aids or drinking alcohol in labor. Some providers suggest marijuana or other drugs for anxiety or pain relief (which might not be legal). These options, and the risks and benefits of each, should be discussed with your provider, ideally before labor so you're best able to make informed choices.

BLADDER CATHETER

Sometimes, because of anesthesia or because of the baby's position, it can be difficult to urinate during labor. Most people with an epidural can't feel the need to urinate and can't mobilize their muscles to empty their bladder. It's common for a nurse to thread a thin flexible tube through your urethra into your bladder to drain your urine. In some cases, this catheter will be left in place, secured with tape to the side of your leg and attached to a urine collection bag. It can be left in place for the rest of labor and removed during pushing. In other cases, a nurse will reinsert every few hours, as needed, to drain your bladder. The decision to leave it in place or repeatedly catheterize you is usually a policy of the birthing location, and you can find out in advance what is typical at your birth location. There is a small risk of infection from the catheter in your bladder. Some people also experience discomfort when the catheter is placed and mild discomfort while the catheter is in.

While bladder catheters are common in hospitals with epidurals, they're also used in birth centers and at home less frequently. Several times I've been with clients laboring at home without any pain medication who could not empty their bladder. The position of their baby's head seemed to be blocking their ability to pee. After hours of not being able to void, their midwives used a catheter to drain their (very full) bladder and give them some relief. Astrid, for example, went hours and hours without being able to pee during her homebirth and was struggling to progress beyond 5 cm. Her midwife inserted a catheter, and an enormous amount of urine came out, much to her relief. Less than two hours later she gave birth. Her full bladder was likely making it harder for the baby to move lower, slowing labor progress. This small intervention made an enormous difference for her labor.

BREAKING THE WATER—ARTIFICIAL RUPTURE OF MEMBRANES

As I mentioned in the previous chapter, the amniotic sac attached to your placenta fills with fluid that cushions and protects the baby during pregnancy. Providers in all birth locations, on occasion, will recommend breaking your amniotic sac and releasing the water. It's most common with doctors in hospitals, but midwives in birth centers and at home also do this sometimes.

When a provider breaks your water, they use a tool called an amniohook. Often people describe this tool as similar to a crochet hook or a knitting needle. I think this description makes having your water broken sound both scarier and more painful than it is. I wouldn't want a knitting needle in my vagina, even if they look somewhat similar! I describe the amniohook as a small plastic wand with a small curve on one end. Much like a cervical exam, your provider will insert two fingers into your vagina to feel your cervix and the bag of water. They guide the amniohook in, make a small opening in the membrane, and release the water.

Some people imagine releasing the water as a onetime event, but your water will continue to leak through the rest of labor. If the leaking bothers you, you may want to wear a pad or keep a towel between your legs.

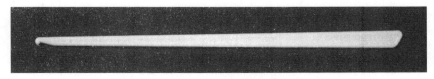

Amniohook, a plastic tool used for breaking the water.

Breaking the water might be suggested to help labor progress, or it might be recommended when placing an internal monitor. There are risks to breaking the water, primarily an increased risk of infection if there's a long time between rupturing the membranes and giving birth. In my own first labor I consented to having my water broken when I was 9 cm, and my son was born within about an hour. The risk of infection in this scenario was incredibly low. I have, however, been with clients when a provider was considering breaking the water very early in labor, at 1–2 cm for example, and the risk of infection is higher in this case.

OTHER POSSIBLE MEDICATIONS

There is a wide variety of other medications that might be offered or used during labor; this is not an exhaustive list. For example, medications can be offered to counter heartburn (like Tums, Pepcid, Bicitra) or to stop vomiting (Zofran, Diclegis); to assist with sleeping in early labor; to raise your blood pressure if it drops too low (often epinephrine) or lower your blood pressure if it's too high (magnesium citrate, among others); or, especially if you already have a prescription for it, antianxiety medications might be available. If your contractions are too frequent and your baby is distressed by it, they might want to stop contractions (often with terbutaline). If your contractions are not frequent enough, it's common to give medication to make them more frequent (usually Pitocin, see chapter 11). If you have concerns or questions about what medications might be available, recommended, or used during labor, ask your provider.

ENEMAS

An enema is most commonly used to relieve constipation by inserting a tube into your rectum, introducing fluid (often water, sometimes oil) into your bowels, and flushing out stool. While enemas were once common in hospitals for laboring people, they're no longer common. That said, enemas can be useful for stimulating labor, relieving intense pressure if you're constipated and contracting, and clearing out stool if you are anxious about the possibility of pooping while pushing. The downside of an enema can be discomfort when you get it and, for some people, forceful discharge of your bowels immediately afterward. Speak with your provider about the availability of enemas at your birth location and their use. If enemas are not available already, speak with them about buying your own enema kit at a pharmacy and using it during labor if desired.

ASSISTED VAGINAL DELIVERY

There are a couple of ways a doctor can assist with a vaginal delivery including a vacuum extractor (ventouse) or forceps. These technologies are suggested when you are fully dilated, your baby is low in the birth canal, your provider believes they can be born vaginally, and continuing to push without assistance is not recommended. This might mean that the baby is showing signs of distress (usually certain types of decelerations in their heart rate), you have pushed for a long time and are either too exhausted to continue or your pushing efforts are no longer moving the baby down, or you have a medical condition that makes more pushing less safe (like a heart problem).

The primary reason to consider an assisted vaginal delivery is to avoid a Cesarean birth. An assisted vaginal delivery might be preferable to a Cesarean birth because it can be done more quickly, it doesn't involve major surgery and the risks associated with that, it is often easier to heal from (although not always), and it's usually safer to have a vaginal delivery for those planning to have more children (again, not always).

A vacuum extractor is a plastic disc or cup that's placed on the top of your baby's head. There is a vacuum pump that allows a doctor to suction the disc to your baby's head and a handle for your doctor to pull on while you push, helping guide your baby out vaginally. Forceps look like two large spoons or tongs, and they're placed on either side of your baby's head inside your vagina. They are similarly used by a doctor to pull your baby while you push, guiding them through the birth canal and a vaginal delivery.

These technologies have been around for a long time—obstetric forceps were likely invented in the 1600s. There are many types of forceps often used for delivering babies in different positions. For your purposes, the most useful thing to know is that they're incredibly uncommon, and it's always up to you whether you want to consent to their use. Assisted vaginal delivery was much more common in the US decades ago, but the rate of assisted vaginal births is now 3 percent,[19] and the vast majority of those are vacuum extraction. With the rising popularity of vacuums starting in the 1950s, many providers aren't even trained to use forceps any longer.

With an assisted vaginal delivery, there's a small increase in the risk of more serious damage to your vagina, perineum, and anus[20] from increased tearing and/or the use of episiotomy (see below). There's also a slight risk of complications for the baby, including damage to their scalp, nerve problems, and bleeding inside the skull.[21] In teaching hospitals where residents regularly assist as part of their training, it's common for a resident to place and pull the vacuum.

You might want to ask how much experience they have with vacuum assistance and decide if you'd prefer your OB or another OB perform this procedure. You should also speak with the doctor who has recommended an assisted vaginal delivery more about these risks and any concerns you have. In some cases you may feel that an assisted vaginal delivery is preferable and consent to a vacuum or forceps; in other cases you may feel the risks are too high and opt for a Cesarean birth instead.

EPISIOTOMY

An episiotomy is a surgical incision made in your perineum and vagina to enlarge the opening your baby is coming through during a vaginal birth. This is usually performed with surgical scissors and local numbing medication, and the area is then stitched closed after your baby is born. I've never met anyone who didn't instinctively want to avoid an episiotomy, but it's an intervention that might be preferable in specific moments.

Episiotomies were incredibly common in the US for a long time, but they are thankfully less common now (although still above the recommended level). In 1996 the World Health Organization recommended that the episiotomy rate should be approximately 10 percent or less, and the routine use of episiotomies is no longer recommended by any medical organization.[22] Yet in 2012 it was still one of the most common medical procedures, at about 12 percent of vaginal births countrywide, with some providers still performing episiotomies at rates of 30 or 40 percent of the time.[23] In my own practice, I've seen a rate closer to 4 percent. If your provider still performs routine episiotomies or has a rate above 10 percent, you may want to switch to a provider with a lower rate.

There are two types of episiotomies: median and mediolateral. If you imagine your vulva like a clock, with your urethra and clitoris at noon and your perineum and anus at six o'clock, a median episiotomy is a cut directly down toward six o'clock, and a mediolateral episiotomy is an incision to the side, at closer to five o'clock or seven o'clock. A mediolateral episiotomy has much fewer risks associated with it.

Routine episiotomies are not recommended because they increase complications without benefits. For a long time, the common argument in favor of episiotomies was ease of repair and improved wound healing, but this isn't true. There are no long-term benefits of episiotomies for healing. Episiotomies don't protect the pelvic floor and might weaken the pelvic floor. Further, episiotomies often create larger wounds. Studies say median episiotomy wounds are about

3 cm longer than a tear and median episiotomies are also associated with as much as four times the risk of the most severe types of perineal damage (unlike mediolateral episiotomies).[24]

That said, there are some circumstances where, despite these risks, there are benefits to considering an episiotomy. The most common reason to consider an episiotomy is to speed up delivery when your baby shows signs of serious distress. An episiotomy can speed up delivery by several minutes, helpful for a very distressed baby if other efforts haven't worked and delivery is only blocked by perineal tissue. Sometimes an episiotomy will be performed to help when placing forceps or a vacuum, but there's no reason to do this routinely as it's often unnecessary. Under these circumstances, a median episiotomy is especially risky, tripling the risk of injury to the anus.

In finding a provider, you may want to ask about their use of episiotomies: how often they perform them, for what reasons, and which type they perform. Because episiotomies are usually done in the last minutes before a baby is born, you should anticipate that your ability to make a choice about an episiotomy and give consent to the procedure might be compromised. You may also want to make sure that your provider will discuss an episiotomy with you before performing one. I have been present during several births where a care provider used confusing language to discuss their intention to perform an episiotomy— such as "I am just going to make a little space" or "I am going to make a little more room for your baby"—and my client would not have understood what they were agreeing to had I not clarified. Working with a provider you trust, who only performs this intervention when absolutely needed, is important if you want to avoid an unnecessary episiotomy.

CONTROLLING POSTPARTUM BLEEDING, PREVENTING HEMORRHAGE

After your baby is born, you'll still need to deliver your placenta, and your provider will want to carefully monitor your blood loss. Postpartum hemorrhage (PPH) is the leading cause of death during pregnancy, and your provider will want to ensure you do not hemorrhage and, if you do, that you get swift treatment to control the bleeding and restore your health.

There's a good amount of bleeding involved with every labor and delivery. Many people are surprised by the amount of bleeding, even when assured it's normal. I had been incorrectly led to believe that my postpartum bleeding would be similar to a heavy period and was shocked.

One of the primary sources of this bleeding is from the wound inside your uterus left by the placenta. The placenta is attached to your uterine wall, and after it has been expelled, there is a big open wound left inside your uterus. Your uterus should contract after the placenta is gone, shrinking and tightening, reducing the placenta wound and slowing the flow of blood. You might also bleed from an episiotomy, a vaginal laceration, or from a Cesarean incision. Properly controlling bleeding from any of these wounds and prompt suturing is important for minimizing blood loss postpartum.

Many providers, especially in hospitals, recommend the routine use of synthetic oxytocin (Pitocin) postpartum to cause more contractions and reduce bleeding. There are known factors that increase the risk of a PPH that can be anticipated before giving birth, such as giving birth to twins or multiples, having a very large baby (macrosomia), and induction of labor (especially long inductions where large amounts of Pitocin have been given). That said, people with no risk factors can have a PPH. Routinely giving everyone postpartum Pitocin is an evidence-based practice for reducing the frequency of PPH, and this may be your provider's standard of care.[25]

After you birth the placenta, you'll likely experience a fair amount of uncomfortable pressing on your belly to feel your uterus and make sure it's firm. Your provider or nurses will check your pads to see how much you're bleeding, and it's common to also check your blood pressure as a tool for monitoring blood loss.

In addition to postpartum Pitocin and manually massaging your uterus, there are a variety of interventions and medications (collectively called uterotonic drugs) that can be used to increase contractions and reduce bleeding. Medications such as Methergine and Cytotec, among others, are usually on hand in hospitals and often in out-of-hospital births too. They can be given as a shot into your muscle (Methergine) or pills inserted rectally (Cytotec). Some midwives also will give their clients herbal tinctures or have them eat some of the placenta to control a PPH. You should speak with your provider about what medications and interventions they routinely use to prevent and manage PPH. Especially for people giving birth out of hospital, it's important to know what will be available. Transferring to a hospital is not necessarily a quick process, so other methods for controlling bleeding should be available.

CONCLUSION

It's not uncommon for people to find birth plan templates online and come to me with questions about uncommon interventions in the hospital, such as routine enemas, having their pubic hair shaved, or being forced to deliver in an operating room with their legs strapped in stirrups. While all these things were common when my mother gave birth, they're very uncommon now. I've only ever seen pubic hair shaved at the site of the Cesarean incision, for example, and only when a Cesarean birth is happening, not as a precaution. Enemas are often available, and you could certainly ask for one, but no one will be forcing you to have one. Hospitals largely use labor/delivery/recovery (LDR) rooms now, so you can labor, push, deliver, and recover for a few hours in the same place. Stirrups might be attached to your labor bed, and you can ask your provider how or when they use them.

If these possible medications, monitors, and interventions feel overwhelming to you, you might want to return to the chapter on doulas (chapter 7) and consider what having an advocate would look like for you in your birth. A doula should be well trained in what all these interventions are, the pros and cons of each, and how common they are among local providers and birth locations. They should also be able to help you navigate your options without any agenda about your choice to use or refuse any of these interventions.

Some interventions are standard procedure in some locations and may be presented as not optional. Remember, it's your right to consent to, or refuse, any treatment you don't want. You're ultimately in control and get to choose what happens, who does it, and when it happens.

INTERVENTION
PREFERENCES

- What type of **monitoring** should I expect? Intermittent? Continuous?
- Will a **hep lock** be required? Will **IV fluids** be required?
- Are **antibiotics** recommended for me? When will these be administered?
- Are there any other **medications** you expect I might need? How often do you use **Pitocin** and in what circumstances? What about prescription medications I take?
- Are there **TENS machines** available or if I bring my own, can I use it? Do you offer **sterile water injections**? What other labor-coping tools are available?
- Is **nitrous oxide** available?
- Are IV or IM **narcotics** available?
- If I would like an **epidural**, is that available? How long should I expect to wait for an anesthesiologist when I am in labor?
- Is a **bladder catheter** required if I have an epidural? Will it stay in place or will I be catheterized every few hours during labor?
- Do you usually recommend **breaking the water** at some stage of labor if it has not broken already? If I want to refuse, are you comfortable with that?
- Do you assist vaginal delivery with **forceps**? A **vacuum**? Will you perform this procedure yourself, and, if not, who will perform it? Can we talk about the risks and benefits of assisted vaginal delivery versus a Cesarean birth?

- How often do you perform an **episiotomy**? Are there circum-stances where you would recommend it (and what are they)? What type of episiotomy do you perform?
- How common are **Cesarean births** in your practice? When would you recommend one? Do you offer gentle or family-centered Cesareans? (See chapter 14 for more on this.)
- Can you describe what I should expect postpartum? Postpartum **Pitocin**? Other medications? **Sutures**? **Monitoring**?

10

BIRTH PLANS AND LABOR-COPING STRATEGIES

You're likely hearing from friends, family, neighbors, doctors, strangers (or all of the above!) that you shouldn't make plans for your birth because things don't go as planned. Perhaps you've heard people remind you that your baby's health is most important and you must stay flexible. Maybe you have been told that your only plan should be "healthy baby, healthy mommy" (a common phrase I've come to hate, even while I hope you and your baby are both healthy). These warnings are often about preparing you for negative experiences rather than feeling empowered to have a positive experience. Making a birth plan should have the opposite effect. Having a birth plan shouldn't set you up for disappointment or a sense of failure; rather, a plan should be about helping you control the elements that are controllable, make choices that resonate with your desires, and understand what to expect, including how things might change.

I think making plans for childbirth is akin to planning travel adventures. My family travels often, and our trips are among my favorite things. We pick new places each year—Iceland, the Outer Banks, the Grand Canyon, Oregon, Scotland, the Canadian Rockies, Maine, Newfoundland, Kentucky, Tuscany—and there's lots of unpredictability. Yet I book airline tickets even though flights are sometimes canceled or changed, delayed, or overbooked. I reserve hotel rooms and rental housing even though we have occasionally been disappointed by the quality or cleanliness of the place (that musty houseboat in the Netherlands, for example). We make plans even with the small possibility of being let down, because making plans ultimately helps reduce the chances of having those disappointing experiences and really increases the chances of positive experiences.

For my family, the research we do for our vacations and the plans we make ahead of time are absolutely part of what makes the vacations pleasurable. We know ourselves and what we like from our experiences, and how this might differ from what other people might enjoy. My brother loves to vacation at everything-included resorts with restaurants and staff; we prefer off-the-beaten-path rural rental houses. Neither my brother nor I is right or wrong, but each of us is happier for having gone on the adventure that matches our preferences.

Making plans for childbirth helps ensure you have as positive an experience as possible. Sometimes plans need to be altered. Sometimes the plan is to wait and see what you want in the moment. Being able to embrace change and alter the plans is valuable, but that doesn't mean you should abandon plan-making altogether. It makes sense to have hopes and desires, to make choices, and to articulate preferences. It makes sense to plan with all of that in mind.

Childbirth is unpredictable, it's true. But much of what people are warning against is actually quite predictable. If your doctor has the highest Cesarean birthrate in town and you don't want a Cesarean birth, this is a great opportunity to consider the plans you've made and the choices you have. That said, if you are planning a Cesarean birth, this same doctor might be an excellent match. If you'd like to avoid an epidural and have picked a hospital that offers other labor-coping options such as nitrous oxide, access to tubs or showers, and lots of mobility, then you can be assured that you've made a plan that matches your desires.

You *do* have control over some elements of childbirth, and the plans made leading up to birth are important. The process of thinking through your options and making plans can help you make better choices and set yourself up for success—whatever that means for you. In what follows, I aim to help you make plans that match your desires, prepare for the possibility of your plans changing, and think through labor-coping strategies that will work for you.

A huge part of making plans for your birth is the choices you make prenatally. Picking a provider and location helps set the stage for having a birth that matches your expectations. Several years ago I interviewed experienced doulas throughout the country, asking what they do with clients that they believe helps improve birth experiences.[1] As I mentioned before, the clinical data on doulas shows significant improvements for both parents and babies, but the data doesn't explain *how* or *why* these improvements are made. One consistent response from doulas: they help clients make plans. One doula said she believes, even before the birth, she helps improve outcomes by redirecting them to providers who are evidence based and more likely to help them have the birth they're hoping for. She said, "I give a checklist of detailed questions for them to

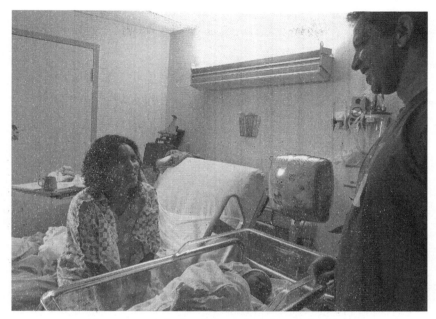

New parents enjoying their newborn hours after birth.

ask their doctors, so they know exactly what their doctors' practices are, so they know if they're trying to get Chinese food at a Kosher deli."

You can want whatever you want, make whatever choices match your preferences, and do whatever you need to do. It's not about the specifics of the birth plan you are making but, instead, about the process of making the plan and figuring out what you'd like from this experience. Recently I visited someone who had a planned homebirth and was nursing her baby in bed when I arrived. The same day, I visited another client who was planning to give birth in the hospital with an epidural and hated the idea of breastfeeding. Guiding them each through the process of making prenatal choices was exactly the same, even if their desires and decisions were different.

I like to assume almost nothing about what my clients might want or need in their labor and birth, although I take as a given that everyone wants to be safe and healthy with a healthy baby. This is the minimum requirement. Beyond this, I ask everyone, "What does your best-case scenario look like? If everything goes perfectly in your childbirth, what happens?" While people often initially answer with a joke, perhaps unprepared to really articulate what they want, valuable conversations follow.

Having a baby is big. You might be confronting the unknowns of birthing your first baby or managing fears or disappointments from a previous experience. It can be confusing, intense, or intimidating to talk about your hopes, fears, and ideas about what a positive birth experience would look like. Many of my clients have been told what they *should* want, fear, or reject (and often in contradictory ways). My client was getting on the train the other day, and the woman who offered her a seat, noticing her belly, casually told her without any previous conversation, "Get the epidural. Seriously, just do it." Later that day she had a business meeting with a client who runs a major corporation. He, equally casually, told her that his wife had used mantras and medication to get through labor without drugs and that she should do the same because it is much better for the baby.

It can be overwhelming to peel back those layers of advice, information, and expectations to figure out what you want from your experience (not just what others tell you to want), but this is how you get at your individual desires and craft a tailored plan. You can think about *why* you want what you want, make choices about your own birth, and make plans that honor what's important to you, not just what you've been told to want.

Good birth plans make for good births. It's true that occasionally having a healthy birth might mean changing some of your plans—an unwanted Cesarean birth might become needed and welcomed even, a homebirth might become too risky and require transfer to the hospital, your blood work might confirm that the epidural you wanted is not safe—but even when plans change, knowing your preferences can help you negotiate the new choices you need to make.

A good birth plan helps you make choices in advance that match your hopes and desires. It can help you know what to expect. It helps prevent spending time during your birth in conflict or disappointed because what you want isn't available. It helps you communicate with other people who'll be assisting you during birth: birth partners, care providers, nurses, assistants. While it might be partially a plan you write down—and I recommend you do (using the worksheet that follows this chapter as a model)—it's also a conversation.

Making a birth plan can help you have conversations in advance about what you'd like and what's possible. Thinking through options ahead of time can help if you're faced with changes to your plans during labor. In making your birth plan, it might be valuable to talk with your support people about your decision-making process: Are you prone to following your instincts or more of a researcher? Do you struggle with decision-making or feel very confident? Think about how you might feel if you needed to negotiate plan changes or are faced with rapid decision-making. How can your support people help you?

When I ask clients to talk through their best-case scenario, I'm certainly not promising that they'll get the exact birth they describe (and people change what they want routinely). Making space to have preferences and think through options is critical, and the conversations we have help people articulate what's most important to them. For example, when I helped Jada and Xavier have their first baby, Jada was very clear in our initial conversations that she wanted an unmedicated vaginal birth. She took an eight-week childbirth education class and learned a wide variety of labor-coping techniques. When we talked about what her best-case scenario looked like, we focused on how she wanted to feel and what she wanted the experience to be like. Jada explained that she wanted to avoid an epidural because she wanted to feel present in her birth and worried that the pain medication would make her feel outside the process.

When labor began, I joined Jada in her apartment and we spent a day and a night laboring together. She lay in her bed while I massaged her back, she took hot showers, we did lunges on the stairs, Xavier made her plates of scrambled eggs to keep her strength up, and we breathed with her through contractions. About twenty hours into it, just after the sun came up, we walked three blocks down crowded Manhattan streets to the hospital. Several well-meaning people stopped to offer us help or let us know there was a hospital nearby, providing some much-needed laughter. At the hospital, she was thrilled to hear she was 7 cm dilated. After fetal monitoring, a blood draw, establishing IV access, answering some questions, and being admitted into a labor room, Jada was back to laboring in the shower.

For the next few hours Jada labored on the toilet, in the shower, and on the bed. She became increasingly distant and internal. Back in the shower, she was leaning on the handrail three feet from me but seemed a thousand miles away. I asked her, "What is going on in your head?" She started crying and said she was imagining giving birth and sending the baby to the nursery so she could sleep. "I hate the idea of being in labor, but I hate the idea of the baby being born too. I want to be done so I can sleep." Our prenatal conversations returned to me. Jada wanted to avoid an epidural in order to feel present. She wanted to meet her baby in a joyful way.

Clearly we'd departed from her plan to feel present and joyful, and I was concerned. We talked about options for shifting how she was feeling, and her conclusion was that a nap was the only thing she could see helping her. Unfortunately, she could not lie down or rest her body with the contractions, so napping felt impossible to her. I told her she was doing an excellent job managing her contractions, and I didn't want to undermine her desire to avoid an epidural, so perhaps it made sense for us to talk about what that option would look like for her. After much conversation, she opted for the epidural, napped for a couple of hours, and woke up ready to push. When Jada's son was placed on her chest, she was thrilled. Talking afterward, she was clear she'd made the best decision. While her plan had been to forgo an epidural, she found the change of plans helped her achieve a more important piece of her plan—feeling present and connected to her birth.

Jada had moved from a place of managing pain to suffering: a distinction I often make with clients. While the dictionary definitions of both pain and suffering point to each other (pain is something you suffer, suffering is a type of pain), I think it's useful to isolate the experience of physical pain from the broader experience of suffering when thinking about coping with labor.

In labor you'll likely experience pain from contractions (although some people do not experience these sensations as pain or opt not to use the word "pain" to describe the feelings they have). You might feel cramping or aching in your lower belly, back, pelvis, and hips. These are sensations in your body you might be able to breathe through, move with, ignore, medicate, or otherwise cope with. These sensations are temporary, both because contractions happen with breaks between them (you'll actually spend most of your labor in those spaces in between) and because labor always ends. In labor, having multiple strategies for managing these physical sensations is key.

Suffering might be caused by physical pain, especially when your coping strategies aren't working and need to be shifted, but, to me, it's also about the larger emotional experience. Pain in labor is something you can cope with. It has a purpose. It's work that's being done. But if you have moved from pain to suffering, like Jada had in the final hours of her labor, you might need to take actions to transform your experience, alleviate the suffering, and move back into a place where you're able to have a more positive experience of your birth. This might mean you get an epidural like Jada did, or have a talk with someone to shift your emotional experience, change your position or rest your body in a needed way, or move into new coping strategies that bring you back to a more tolerable place.

Your plan need not be grounded in specific choices—although it certainly can be—because how you'd like to *feel* is important. Your plan might address questions like:

What will make you feel safe?
What will help you feel in control?
What will help you feel supported?
When you need to make choices, how would you like to approach that?

Who do you want with you?
How do you imagine feeling comforted in labor?
What strategies will you use to cope with labor?
What happens if you've moved from pain to suffering?
If plans need to change, how will you approach those changes?

COPING STRATEGIES FOR LABOR

Many childbirth methods suggest that everyone can successfully navigate labor with the same tools and techniques. In my experience, we all cope differently. What helps us feel calm and capable is not one size fits all. Thankfully, you did not just arrive in your body during this pregnancy—you likely have years and years of learning how you cope with things like pain, fear, exhaustion, stress, or anxiety. You already have coping strategies you use in your day-to-day life, so you don't necessarily need to learn entirely new ways of being in your body. Tapping into your coping strategies and adapting them to the challenges of labor is the task.

When I ask clients about their birth plans, I ask a series of questions about how they've managed pain, stress, or anxiety during their lives. I ask these questions to help identify what coping strategies they're already using and how those might (or might not) work in labor:

In what ways are you preparing for this labor and birth?
What do you anticipate will be your greatest challenge while in labor?
What do you anticipate will be your greatest source of strength in labor?
Some people find labor challenging or painful. In previous challenging or uncomfortable situations (sickness, headache, stress), what methods have you used to comfort yourself?
Some people might find the intensity of labor scary or they get anxious. When frightened or anxious, what techniques do you use to regain your calm?
If it is useful for you, describe an image, place or experience that, if referenced while in labor, could help to soothe and center you as needed.
In what ways do you hope my support will be helpful to you? What types of assistance do you imagine will be most useful? What about the help you imagine will be useful from other members of your birth team (your family, partner, friends, or whoever you have opted to have support you)?

I ask these questions because, ultimately, no matter what your plans are for childbirth, coping strategies are essential and they vary enormously from person to person. Identifying what yours are and how they might be used in labor is critical.

When I met with Elizabeth, she explained that her first birth experience hadn't gone how she'd hoped. Before giving birth to her first baby, she hadn't worried about preparing because, as she said, "My whole plan was to have an epidural." Unfortunately, a crowded hospital meant it took twelve hours to get an epidural. Then the epidural was not working well and she was progressing quickly, so her doctor refused her more medication for fear it would hinder her ability to push. She labored and birthed with little pain relief and without any other prepared coping strategies. Her husband felt lost and unprepared to help, and they both recalled the experience negatively.

During that meeting, our goal was to talk through what happened last time and how Elizabeth (and her husband) could prevent the same thing from happening again. This meant, in part, that we talked about strategies for making sure she got to the hospital in time to get pain medication, and that she was able to advocate for more immediate admission instead of being sent to walk the halls like last time. It also meant talking through coping strategies like breathing, massage, movement, and positioning to use before getting pain medication. I coached her husband through breathing, and we talked through managing the long drive to their hospital when he'd be focused on the road. Elizabeth did well with guided meditations for stress, she told me, so we found a few she could play in the car. We talked through what her husband might say to help her stay calm—she liked the idea of being reminded she's strong and capable. Our strategizing and preparation focused on ensuring she didn't feel out of control again and that they had strategies beyond the epidural.

The next day I met with Simone; her goal was very much to avoid having an epidural during her birth. Her question for me: "What should I be doing to prepare myself physically and emotionally for what labor is going to be like?" She was aware from friends' stories and popular culture that labor would likely be one of the most difficult experiences of her life, and she worried her previous coping strategies (eating cereal, listening to romance novels on audiobooks, getting massages, and taking baths, she told me) might not work well.

Simone and I spent our time together talking about what to expect in labor— the signs and stages and likely experiences—and how her established coping strategies could translate into labor-coping tools. While she might or might not like bowls of cereal in labor, staying hydrated is important, so focusing on hydration could be useful. Distraction, perhaps in the form of an audiobook or

TV or even her partner speaking to her, might be helpful. We practiced labor massage techniques, and I taught her partner how to squeeze her hips and press on her lower back in ways she liked. Taking baths, or showers, are a common labor-coping tool and would likely help her relax. Her familiar strategies translated nicely for labor, building her confidence.

I share these interactions with Simone and Elizabeth to highlight that, no matter what the plan is, having both mental and physical coping strategies is important. Coping strategies can differ vastly, but they should never be singular. Elizabeth's entire plan for her first birth had been to get an epidural; that plan failed her. For her second birth, she was clear she needed more strategies even as she still hoped to get relief from an epidural. She ultimately used several strategies when she had her daughter: the nonmedical techniques helped her get to the hospital and stay calm while she waited for an epidural, her husband was prepared to be more forceful in their advocacy for an epidural right away, and the epidural worked well to help her relax through the rest of labor. Simone worried that her previous strategies would not serve her well, but in conversation we were able to think about her strategies and practice for labor. When she went into labor, showering, pacing her apartment, and tons of massage helped her manage labor without an epidural as she hoped.

I remind clients often that you don't become someone other than yourself when you are in labor. Tapping into the strategies that already resonate with you are most effective for coping with labor. I once supported someone who had the lights off, a season's worth of cooking shows on mute, a soundtrack of instrumental versions of love songs from the nineties, and she was breathing, moaning, and swaying her way through an induction with Pitocin. This worked for her. Similarly, I've seen people cope with labor by singing show tunes through contractions, squeezing someone's hand, playing Scrabble, watching hockey and basketball, dancing to Lady Gaga, chanting (sometimes even chanting curse words), or going internal with things like a face mask or sunglasses and earplugs to tune everything else out. When clients ask me about various childbirth methods and what works the best, I am quick to point out that I don't believe any of them work universally. We are not one size fits all. I prefer to talk through your *current* coping strategies and use those as a guide for thinking about the techniques that might be ideal for you.

Several years ago, Rachael told to me that getting hot triggers panic attacks in her. She was planning a homebirth, where tubs are common, but soaking in a tub would likely make her hot. Rachael said she thrives on movement, likes to work out when stressed or in pain, and does well with being given directions. In both of her labors, these were the strategies that helped her have great experiences. She stayed mobile throughout, preferring upright positions, pacing the house, and powering through contractions with lunges and squats. When she lost focus or started struggling, I stepped in with concrete suggestions, moved with her, and used massage to relax her between contractions. This worked perfectly for Rachael.

Yet these strategies might work terribly for someone who prefers quiet, dark, calm, and restful spaces when working through challenges. For that person, supported side-lying positions with pillows in bed, quiet music or meditations, candles or no light, a hot bath, and little or no talking might be ideal. This was the case for Lee who gave birth to her daughter last year after hours of only wanting to lie on her side without being touched or spoken to. Her wife and I stayed quietly nearby offering sips of water, reminding her to breathe with our breath, and helping her to the restroom periodically. Even when pushing, she stayed on her side with her eyes closed. These strategies worked perfectly for her.

Labor is often compared to running a marathon. I disagree. Giving birth is not like running a marathon, even if it might be a similarly challenging experience. Running a marathon is something few people ultimately do. It usually requires months of training and takes specific types of physical capacities to complete. That is not the case with birth. Birth doesn't require the athleticism of a marathon. Preparing for birth requires thinking through what you want and don't want, both clinically and how you want to feel, and tapping into your coping strategies.

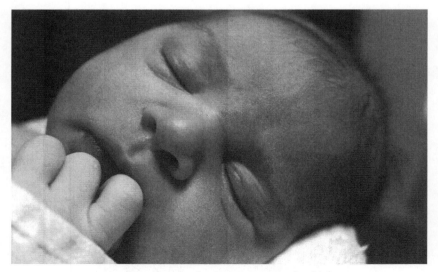

Newborn sleeping in a parent's arms after birth.

PREPARING A BIRTH PLAN

The internet overflows with funny takes on the birth plan—from dolphin-assisted water birth jokes to requests for the nonlaboring partner to be given drugs during labor. You might also find advice to skip a birth plan all together. I disagree. For people birthing in hospitals in particular, I think a well-crafted birth plan is a gift to the hospital staff because it makes their jobs easier. Below are the components I think are key to making a great birth plan to share with nurses at the hospital.

Identify yourself and your team: Put your name in bold on the top of the page with your date of birth. Below this, list your husband/wife/coparent/partner if you have one. Follow this with the name of your provider, your doula or any other support people, and your chosen pediatrician. Include your address and your phone numbers. It might look like this:

- **Erika Jackson (DOB: July 6, 1984)**
- **Husband:** Allen Jackson
- **Doctors:** Westside Doctor Group
- **Doula:** Megan Davidson
- **Sister:** Pam Smith
- **Pediatrician:** Happy Kids Pediatrician Group
- **Address:** 275 N Main St. Apt 12, City, State
- **Cell:** 555-111-1234 (Erika), 555-432-0987 (Allen)

Share your pregnancy history: Following this, share your basic pregnancy information to help the staff quickly identify key info about your health and the care you might need. This can include your estimated due date, last menstrual period (or IVF transfer date), group beta strep status, sex of baby, pregnancy history (all pregnancies including miscarriages and elective terminations), and any complications in this pregnancy (hypertension, gestational diabetes, anemia, etc.). It might look like this:

- **EDD: December 21, 2019**
- **LMP:** March 16, 2019
- **GBS:** negative
- **Sex of baby:** surprise!
- **Pregnancy history:** 1. miscarriage (2017), 2. Current
- **Complications in pregnancy:** gestational diabetes, controlled with diet and exercise

Share your basic medical history: Next it's helpful to share basic health history including height and weight, vaccinations during pregnancy, any chronic health conditions (asthma, heart conditions, diabetes, diseases), surgeries, medications you take, allergies (and your reaction), and if you drink, smoke, or use drugs beyond those prescribed. It might look like this:

- **Height and weight: 5'6", 152 lbs. (pre-pregnancy), 179 lbs. (currently)**
- **Vaccines:** flu vaccine, 10/2019, and TDAP vaccine, 11/2019
- **Health history:** great health. Asthma, triggered by cold weather (inhaler 1–2x yearly)
- **Surgeries:** wisdom teeth (2001), LEEP (2004), shoulder surgery (2013)
- **Medications:** prenatal vitamins, valacyclovir (started at 36 weeks), 2 doses Rhogam
- **Allergies:** penicillin (hives as child)
- **No drinking, no drugs, no smoking**

State your preferences: Finally, finish with a list of preferences for the birth and immediate postpartum. It's great to discuss preferences with your care providers in advance, but the hospital staff will be strangers. Your preferences might include clothing, pain medication, monitoring, IV fluids, mobility, medical students, cord clamping, feeding, separation from your baby, newborn procedures, and your placenta, among other things. You might also want to make reminders about your preferences for pronouns or the names and pronouns of your family/team, about medications you need, or about religious or personal preferences (such as modesty or sex of care providers treating/touching you), for example. It might include statements such as:

PREFERENCES:

- I identify as a man and will be the father of my child. I would like help ensuring everyone who interacts with me from the staff uses appropriate pronouns and titles to refer to me.
- I would like to wear my own clothing during labor.
- I would like to my body to be well covered during labor to maintain my modesty.
- I prefer to only have female nurses and doctors touch me during labor.
- I am aware pain medication is available and prefer not to be offered it.
- I am interested in nitrous oxide during labor.
- I am/am not planning to have an epidural.
- I would like intermittent (or wireless) monitoring and as much mobility as possible.
- I prefer not to have IV fluids during labor.
- I would prefer to have no medical students be involved in my care.
- I would like to delay cord clamping and have my baby skin to skin after the birth.
- My husband/wife/mom/sister/friend would like to cut the umbilical cord.
- I plan to chest/breastfeed or I plan to formula feed and would appreciate help with that.
- We would like to have our baby with us at all times.
- We would prefer to have our baby in the nursery overnight.
- I was given Rhogam in my pregnancy and might need it postpartum.

- We request/decline vitamin K for our baby after birth.
- We request/decline erythromycin eye ointment for our baby.
- We request/decline the hep B vaccine for our baby.
- We are/are not planning to circumcise.
- I would like to take my placenta home with me.

INDUCTIONS, VBACS, TWINS, AND CESAREAN BIRTHS

/

11

INDUCTION OF LABOR

It was one week after her due date when Yael went for a routine prenatal visit at her OB's office. The exam started smoothly, but an ultrasound showed her amniotic fluid was too low. For the baby's sake, her doctor said, she couldn't wait to go into labor on her own. She should be induced that night. Yael was disappointed and nervous. She stood in a cramped hallway, people walking around her awkwardly as she cried on the phone with me. We talked through what to expect, and I reminded her this was still her birth even if the plans had changed.

After a nice meal, Yael and Mark checked in to the hospital for a slow night with little activity. In the morning, Pitocin was started and it worked quickly. By 10:00 a.m. contractions were every three to four minutes, big but not over-whelming. Yael said, "Breathing through them, I still felt like I was in control." At 11:00 a.m. a resident did a cervical exam: 3 cm dilated and 50 percent thinned out. This was progress, and she was happy for it. Contractions continued to get closer and more intense, but at 12:30 p.m. when another doctor examined her, she was still 3 cm and now 80 percent thinned. Yael was freaked out by this news, and I had to remind her this was still progress. The cervical exam had momentarily set her back emotionally.

She was hooked up to monitors and IVs because of the induction. Her mobility was limited, and getting in a shower or tub wasn't an option. Lying down on the bed felt terrible, so she stood next to the bed leaning over it during contractions. By now, contractions were "body wracking and overwhelming," and Yael said each one felt stronger than the last one. In the space between, the pain was gone and she could relax and refocus. In the breaks she sat in a chair, leaning back onto Mark, who stood behind her with a pillow for her head. She'd fall asleep for a minute or two, waking up into another contraction. A couple of hours passed like this before her doctor returned. This time her cervix was 5–6 cm and 100 percent thinned. The doctor told Yael she'd be in labor at least three more hours, suggested she consider an epidural, and left. Yael was devastated. She said three more hours seemed impossible and unbearable.

I disagreed with his estimate and told her so: "No way. He's just throwing out a number. He's wrong." As I helped her off the bed, I said I believed she'd be pushing within an hour. Almost immediately after standing, Yael threw up. In the middle of the vomiting, a huge contraction hit and with it, her water broke. She looked at me, confused and overwhelmed "You're almost there," I told her.

It was too intense for Yael to keep standing, so I guided her onto the bed on her hands and knees. She began to feel the urge to push. Mark was excited, yelling, "This is it! This is it!" I alerted the nurse, who called the doctor back to confirm she was ready to push. Mark put on a song she wanted playing for the birth. I remember hearing it over and over. Mark could see the dark hair on their baby's head, and his enthusiasm was uncontained. As she slid into the doctor's hands, Mark yelled, "It's a girl!"

Yael's birth experience is a nice example of what it can look like to have your labor induced. Induction is defined as the act of causing—in this case, it specifically refers to causing uterine contractions to prompt labor in hopes of a vaginal birth. An induction is usually considered successful when it results in a vaginal birth (within a specific time frame, sometimes twenty-four hours from the time Pitocin is given, sometimes forty-eight hours from the beginning of the induction). Inductions can, and regularly do, also result in a Cesarean birth.

In the last thirty years, the number of inductions has risen from less than 10 percent of births in 1990 to nearly a quarter of births today.[1] Frequency of inductions varies enormously from provider to provider in part because of the types of patients and pregnancies they support (higher risk versus low risk) and in part because of their approach to birth and assessing risk. Some providers routinely induce far more than a quarter of their patients, even twice that, and other providers induce far less than a quarter of their patients. If avoiding an induction is important to you, it'll be valuable for you to question potential providers about their rate of induction.

Given the overall frequency of inductions, it can be valuable for all pregnant people to prepare for the possibility. In what follows, I'll help you make sense of why an induction might be recommended to you as well as times when you might question that recommendation. I'll walk you through what medications or interventions could be used in an induction and the risks and benefits of each (plus the risks and benefits of inductions generally). Finally, I finish with tips and tools for helping you prepare for and navigate an induction if you're having one.

REASONS AN INDUCTION MIGHT BE OFFERED OR RECOMMENDED

Medically recommended inductions are prompted by concerns about the health of your baby or your own health. Typically this means the risks associated with continuing the pregnancy are considered higher than the possible risks associated with more immediate birth, but it's rarely an exact science. How your provider interprets risk is a significant factor.

Usually gestational age (how many weeks pregnant you are) is a primary consideration in evaluating risk versus benefit for recommending an induction. If you've not yet reached full term, your provider might continue to monitor whatever concerns they have for you or your baby while trying to continue the pregnancy. If you're pregnant with one baby, full term is reached at thirty-nine weeks gestation (a week before your estimated due date), and this is considered safest for your baby (unless other risks outweigh the risk of being born early).

If you're already full term, an induction might be recommended immediately if a concern arises, as Yael's birth story exemplified. If you're late term or post-term—usually defined as one or two weeks past your estimated due date—then a routine induction might be recommended by your provider. Many studies have demonstrated increased risks for pregnant people and their babies postterm,[2] so routine inductions are recommended by nearly all providers by forty-two weeks, if not before. If you're curious or concerned about being induced, you should ask potential providers when and why they recommend induction.

The types of health complications that might prompt the recommendation of an induction include chronic hypertension (high blood pressure) or hypertension that developed in the pregnancy, heart disease or other concerns about your heart, clotting problems such as a pulmonary embolism during pregnancy, diabetes (including gestational diabetes, especially if you're taking insulin), preeclampsia (high blood pressure coupled with concerns about other organs, especially your liver and kidneys), ICP/cholestasis (a pregnancy-specific liver condition that affects the flow of bile and causes itching), or a health crisis that requires prompt treatment such as a cancer diagnosis. There might also be medications you're taking that should be closely controlled with birth (such as blood thinners) that could prompt an induction. While the specifics of your health and pregnancy will vary, these are all generally considered evidence-based reasons for an induction. Sometimes your body size might also prompt a provider to recommend induction. If your weight is the only concern, you may want to ask your provider about the evidence to support an induction over waiting for spontaneous labor.

Inductions are also recommended for complications of the pregnancy such as infection, bleeding caused by the placenta beginning to separate from the uterine wall, or like Yael, low amniotic fluid levels. Being dehydrated increases the chances of a low amniotic fluid reading, so staying hydrated is a good strategy for avoiding an induction you might not need.

Concerns for your baby that could prompt an induction include signs of growth restriction, distress, or a health condition that requires specialists during or after the birth. Again, while the specifics of your situation will vary, there's a significant amount of data to support induction in most of these cases. Inductions are also often recommended when your provider suspects your baby is big. Size estimates aren't very accurate at the end of pregnancy, and studies show most suspected big babies are not,[3] making this another situation where, absent other concerns, you might ask your provider for the evidence to support induction.

Another scenario where an induction is often recommended is if your water breaks when you aren't in labor. If this happens before about thirty-four weeks pregnant, your providers might try to delay labor, favoring keeping your baby inside. If this happens beyond about thirty-four weeks, your provider will likely recommend inducing labor. Because there's a higher risk of infection once your water has broken, there is a lot of evidence that it's best to avoid cervical exams in this scenario[4] (they can confirm your water is broken with a swab, so an exam is usually not needed). Studies suggest that induction promptly after your water breaks decreases the time until birth, decreases the rate of infection, and reduces the likelihood of your baby needing to be admitted to the NICU after the birth while not increasing the rate of Cesarean birth.[5] In my practice, I've seen huge variation in how promptly induction is started after the water breaks. This is a good question to ask your provider.

Beyond medical reasons for an induction, some are scheduled for convenience or preference. You might schedule an induction because it gives you a sense of control, it's easier to plan for your older children or support people you want to be with you, or because of work (a military spouse that is being deployed, for example). You might want to schedule it to avoid birthing on a holiday or for religious or cultural reasons. One of my clients, for example, has agreed to interventions in order to have her children born on days that, for spiritual reasons, are preferable for creating harmony in their family. My own mother was not induced, but she refused to push with my brother, holding him in until the clock passed midnight because in 1976, giving birth to her son on Richard Nixon's birthday offended her.

Another reason a non–clinically needed induction might be recommended is for your provider's schedule. If you're working with a large practice, you might prefer to have control over which doctor or midwife is there during your birth. Many providers are available only one or two days a week, and an induction can help control who's with you. Alternatively, an induction might not be your preference, but your provider might recommend it for their convenience or for ease of hospital schedules. This is a situation where you might prefer not to consent to an induction.

INDUCTION TECHNIQUES

Inductions themselves are as varied as the reasons for having an induction. An induction is not one unified experience. Rather, it's a series of possible interventions, used in different ways by different providers, with varied risks and success rates. When I explain inductions to clients, I describe it as similar to the choose-your-own-adventure gamebooks of my youth. It's impossible to predict how your body and your baby will respond so you can't know for certain what the whole plan will be until you are already being induced.

While inductions are unpredictable, there are a lot of things we do know, and I detail that in what follows. There are a few medications that are routinely used (such a Cervidil, Cytotec, and Pitocin), and there are interventions that are very common (such as inserting a balloon catheter into your cervix or breaking your water). Many studies have assessed which medications and interventions, in which order, and under which circumstances produce the best results. I've included much of that information to help you navigate your options and preferences. If an induction is scheduled, or if you want to talk about induction options with a provider, you can ask what they usually recommend and what's available at your birth location.

Two important factors will help decide what medications or interventions might be used to begin your induction. The first is an assessment of your cervix before the induction. Your provider might reference the Bishop score (or cervix score), which is a prelabor scoring system developed by an OB in the 1960s (Dr. Bishop). Using the information gathered from a cervical exam (dilation, effacement, station of the baby, consistency of the cervix, and position of the baby), your provider can calculate a score and predict the chances an induction will end in a vaginal birth. Scores below 5 are less favorable, and scores above 9 are very favorable (but each individual birth is different so your low score could result in a very easy, successful induction or, vice versa). Of note, the Bishop score is less accurate when you've previously given birth vaginally. If you've had a vaginal delivery already, you have an excellent chance of delivering vaginally again, even if your Bishop score is low. Your induction will likely take less time and require fewer interventions. Bishop score calculators can be found online.

The second factor that will help decide which medications or interventions are used at the beginning of your induction is whether you are already contracting (and how frequently). If you're having frequent contractions, even if they're painless and your cervix is not changing, this can limit which medications you can be safely given.

Most inductions begin with a cervical ripener such as Cytotec (misoprostol) or Cervidil (dinoprostone), meant to help soften and thin your cervix. A cervical ripener can significantly improve your Bishop score, increasing the chances your induction will end in a vaginal delivery. If your Bishop score is already high, this step might be skipped.

Cervidil is a vaginal suppository placed near the cervix for ten to twelve hours. Cytotec is a pill, and during inductions it's often given vaginally (placed on the cervix) but it can be used orally (dissolved under the tongue or in your cheek). Both of these medications are hormone-like substances (called prostaglandins) that can cause contractions but aren't expected to alone cause labor (although infrequently this does happen). These medications often make people feel crampy, and the hope is that after one or more doses your cervix will start to soften and thin.

Cytotec is considerably cheaper than Cervidil but isn't currently approved by the FDA for cervical ripening or labor induction (although it's approved in Europe for induction). Cervidil is FDA approved but much more expensive. This can impact which medication is available at your birth location. The data on which method is more effective and safe is a bit contradictory, but generally studies have concluded that using Cytotec is most effective (some suggest it's best administered vaginally, others suggest it's best administered orally).[6] That said, because it's not FDA approved, some hospitals don't stock it. The side effects of using either of these cervical ripeners can include hyperstimulation of your uterus (too many contractions), fever, chills, vomiting, and diarrhea. In my experience, cramping is the most common sensation reported after having either medication administered. Due to the risk of uterine hyperstimulation, these medications are typically only used for induction in hospitals, require monitoring of you and the baby once given, and are not typically given to people who previously had a Cesarean birth. Additionally, these medications are not typically administered if you're having noticeable contractions, because this increases the risk of hyperstimulation.

If you're given a cervical ripener and it hyperstimulates your uterus—usually defined as either more than five contractions in the span of ten minutes, or individual contractions that are lasting longer than two minutes—you may need a medication to counter this. If your baby is tolerating contractions well, your provider may not react quickly to the hyperstimulation. If your baby's heart rate shows signs of distress (typically this means their heart rate slows significantly during or after contractions), terbutaline (often called "terb") might be given. This medication is used in inhalers to help with asthma and is also given as an injection to slow/stop contractions.

In addition to using medications to ripen the cervix, a balloon catheter (also called a cervical balloon, Foley catheter, or Foley balloon) can help mechanically change the cervix during induction. There are two types of these catheters, but they function in nearly the same way, so you'll likely never know the difference. One type, the Foley catheter, is the same tool used to drain your bladder, if needed, and it's stocked routinely in all hospitals. That said, even though it's widely available, some providers aren't well trained in the use of a Foley catheter for cervical ripening and don't use them. Ask your provider if this will be an option available to you.

To insert a balloon catheter, you'll put your feet on stirrups and have a speculum inserted into your vagina and opened so your provider can see your cervix. This will be familiar if you've had routine gynecological exams. Most people don't like this experience both because having a speculum inside of you can be uncomfortable and because the doctor inserting the balloon often has you lie down on an upside-down bedpan under your lower back/butt to make seeing your cervix easier. This position tends to be hard, especially while nine months pregnant.

A thin flexible piece of tubing with a deflated balloon on the end of it is threaded into your cervix (being a little dilated or soft already can help significantly with this). I work in a number of large teaching hospitals where this task of threading the catheter into your cervix is largely done by residents and students. If you're birthing in a similar place, it's OK to ask the person who will be inserting the catheter how experienced they are with the procedure (and request that someone more experienced place it). Since it's not always easy to insert the catheter, especially if this is your first birth, it can take less time and be less painful if the person inserting it is more experienced and confident.

Once inside your cervix, the balloon is inflated with water (injected into the tubing that's outside of your body) and rests in the space between the amniotic sac (or your baby's head if your water is already broken) and the bottom of your uterus. The tubing is then secured to the inside of your thigh with tape, usually with resistance to help "tug" on the catheter. Periodically a nurse, midwife, or doctor might tug on the tubing and retape it tighter (if it doesn't come out). If the balloon comes out, this typically means your cervix is more open, usually at least 3 cm. If the balloon has not come out within ten to twelve hours, many providers will opt to remove it at that point.

While the balloon catheter rarely causes labor by itself, it has a good track record for helping your cervix become more favorable for other induction methods and it doesn't have the risk of hyperstimulation associated with the prostaglandins described above. Because of this, it's usually considered safe for people who've had a previous Cesarean birth to be induced with a balloon catheter. Some providers will even use this induction technique without admitting you to the hospital.

Some providers use cervical ripening methods sequentially, giving you a prostaglandin and then once that's worn off, inserting a cervical balloon. This might be the case if the first attempt to insert the balloon failed because the catheter couldn't yet be threaded through the cervix. This is also more common if there isn't a lot of change to the cervix after using one of the cervical ripening medications. In some cases, your provider might suggest using a balloon in combination with medications, such as Cytotec. Studies have shown this decreases the overall time until birth without increasing the risk of Cesarean birth or other complications.[7]

If you began the induction with "an unfavorable cervix" (as measured by a low Bishop score), ideally one or several of these cervical ripening methods will be used with success. If your cervix is more ripe (soft, thin, open), then the next part of the induction is more likely to be successful. As I said before, none of these cervical ripening methods typically cause labor on their own (although infrequently they do) and the next step in an induction is usually to begin administering a Pitocin IV, a synthetic form of the hormone oxytocin that's produced in your body. Synthetic oxytocin is the most common and proven induction method for causing the strong, frequent contractions that open the cervix.

Pitocin is given through an IV on an infusion pump that continuously gives a very precise dose. Unlike a pill or a shot, where once you've been given a dose of medication you cannot take it back, the half-life of Pitocin is very short, just a few minutes. This means it's very easy to adjust the amount of medication to match whatever amount works best for you. Different providers and different hospitals use different protocols, and none of the protocols have been subject to studies that would be necessary to say which protocol is most safe or effective.[8] These protocols differ in the starting dose, the period of time between increasing the dose, if Pitocin needs to be continued once active labor has begun, and the maximum safe amount given at a time. Despite these differences, the success rates are very similar.

Regardless of these differences, it's typical to slowly increase the amount of Pitocin over the course of time, monitoring the frequency of the contractions as well as how the baby is tolerating labor. Pitocin will usually be increased until the contractions are two to three minutes apart and then adjusted as needed to maintain that pattern. If you don't have pain medication, you might be feeling strong contractions already, and seeing the nurse increase the Pitocin periodically can be challenging. Yael remembered watching the nurse up her Pitocin and how important it was for her to be "mentally prepared to stay with it and welcome it." Finding a way to embrace that aspect of the induction made it easier for her to ignore the Pitocin pump and focus on managing her contractions and enjoying the spaces between.

I've had clients try to negotiate with providers about not increasing the Pitocin, and while this is certainly a choice you can make for your own body, it might not result in the type of cervical change that will lead to a vaginal birth. Especially for people who'd hoped to avoid as many interventions as possible, all of the interventions of an induction can be very challenging. That said, inductions are meant to help avoid a Cesarean birth, so embracing the induction once you're in it can sometimes be your best path to a vaginal birth.

It's very common for providers to suggest breaking your water at some point during an induction. Studies suggest that having your water break (either on your own or by a provider) greatly increases the likelihood of a successful induction.[9] Some providers recommend doing this early in an induction—as soon as synthetic oxytocin is begun—and others recommend waiting until active labor has begun. No matter when your provider recommends breaking your water, they should check that your baby's head is low enough to prevent their umbilical cord from coming out when the water breaks (a rare emergency). They'll also monitor the baby's heart rate after breaking your water to ensure your baby is tolerating it well.

For people who've already given birth, sometimes breaking the water is incredibly effective in starting labor. Breaking the water is also a useful induction tool for people who've had a previous Cesarean birth. Once your water is broken, there's a risk of infection, so most providers will limit the number of cervical exams, especially if you are still earlier in labor.

There are a few alternatives to all the medical interventions mentioned above, but all have much lower rates of success. For example, nipple stimulation (usually with your own hands, sometimes by a partner or a breast pump) can cause contractions and be used to induce labor if your cervix is already ripe. This might be done at home prior to an induction, or it might be something you do while in the hospital. Having sex and/or having an orgasm can also help induce labor in some people. If this is something you enjoy, it's worth trying before going to the hospital for an induction. An enema can also help stimulate or intensify contractions.

Another possibility, if your cervix is already a little dilated, is having your provider strip or sweep your membranes. To do this, they insert a finger into your cervix and rotate, detaching the fetal membranes from the lower part of your uterus. It's possible, although not probable, that this could prompt labor—studies on membrane sweeping say it doesn't produce clinically significant results,[10] but I have seen some people go into labor shortly after a sweep. It can be uncomfortable, and some providers do it routinely without asking for consent. If you're concerned about this, speak with your provider prior to any cervical exams to make sure they won't sweep the membranes without consent. You should also speak with your provider about possible side effects and risks of a membrane sweep including bleeding and accidentally breaking the water.

I routinely hear from clients about their efforts to put themselves into labor with long walks, a massage, or eating things like pineapple, eggplant, dates, or spicy food. One Brooklyn restaurant makes a baked ziti that is rumored to bring on labor, and I have had many clients try it. There is little harm in trying these techniques (unless you have an allergy or a health concern that makes these unsafe), but there's also little data to suggest they'll induce labor (with the exception of dates, where there is some data that consumption in late pregnancy is associated with fewer labor interventions).[11] Whenever possible, I find patience most effective. Although we are not entirely certain what biologic processes prompt labor to begin spontaneously, there is much speculation that it is the placenta and/or the baby who triggers labor, and not the actions of the pregnant person. That said, if patience isn't possible and an induction is happening, you certainly can try any of these techniques to see if they might nudge the process forward!

Some people also try at home induction methods, and some providers will suggest these techniques, even with questionable evidence about safety. Herbs, castor oil, evening primrose oil, or homeopathic remedies might all be suggested to you by friends, online forums, or your provider. If you haven't already discussed these with your provider, you should talk to them about the potential risks and make sure they're aware you are considering these options. Acupuncture is also a common recommendation, and I've seen it help people have contractions. If this interests you, talk with your provider and/or local acupuncturist about that option.

WAYS TO PREPARE FOR YOUR INDUCTION

Most of my clients are unhappy about being induced and would have preferred spontaneous labor. If you believe an induction is not necessary and you'd like to avoid induction, that's a good time to ask more questions and do your research. If you recognize the value of the induction being recommended to you, then it might be helpful to turn your energy toward readying yourself to have the most positive experience of your birth. For Fay, this meant a favorite meal the night before, clean sheets on her bed to come home to, scheduling for the day her favorite doctor was on call, and reminding herself how excited she was to meet her babies.

It's incredibly common for people to assume that induced labor is faster than spontaneous labor, imagining the medications and tools result in a faster overall experience. This is absolutely not true. Hospitals tend to be slow. You may be there for hours before anything happens. When the induction begins, all of the data and my own experiences confirm that labor usually takes longer during an induction.

When you're scheduled for an induction, you're usually given a time to arrive at the hospital (typically at night, especially if it's your first baby). While this feels like you have an appointment, at a busy hospital you may wait hours before a nurse or a room are available. Because you are not in labor, you're lower priority than patients arriving in labor, and this can add a lot of time to your induction.

Once you've been moved into triage or a labor room, your blood will be taken, an IV catheter will be put in, your temperature and blood pressure will be monitored, your baby's heart rate and any contractions you're already having will be monitored, and you'll be given a cervical exam. This initial cervical exam, coupled with whether you're already having contractions, will help your provider make a plan for which medications or interventions to begin induction with.

This process often requires several staff communicating with each other and gathering supplies as needed. This can be quick or take hours and involve a lot of waiting. Finding ways to entertain yourself, getting rest during long stretches where nothing is happening, and staying in a good mood are important parts of managing the induction experience.

You and your support people should bring things to help make the hospital experience more comfortable: pillows, blankets, music, movies, books, toiletries, drinks, snacks, and cozy clothing, for example. I've often described this process to clients like air travel. You might get to the airport and find your plane is delayed. You may have to entertain yourself for hours in an airport before beginning a long flight. And the flight itself might be long, uncomfortable, and at times, boring. Having ways to entertain yourself and embrace a positive attitude can help when you face travel delays and long flights and will benefit you during an induction also.

It's common for doctors (and to a lesser degree, nurses) to tell you they'll be back in a specific amount of time (a few minutes, an hour, three hours) and for that not to happen. I've been at inductions where a whole day passed without a doctor seeing my client, even with multiple requests to be seen. They often have multiple patients, scheduled surgeries, and emergencies to manage during their shift. You may have to actively remind people about the next steps in the process and be proactive about helping the hospital staff manage your induction. To this end, I recommend keeping track of when things happen. As a doula, I keep a time log when I'm at births, noting down information like when exams happened, what the dilation and effacement were, when a medication was given or stopped, or when the water broke. It is common to have nurses and doctors change shifts during an induction, and I find that I use this log frequently to help remind staff of what has happened and what's been planned going forward.

In busy NYC hospitals, my clients often get neglected for hours. Sometimes staff might frame this as "being patient," but, while I'm a huge fan of patience, in an induction, being neglected isn't the same as having a patient provider. In fact, the most patient providers I know are also among the most attentive and present with their clients. Don't be afraid to ask to see your provider, to ask questions, to check on the time frame for when medications or interventions are likely to happen, and to speak up if your own notes are different from what you hear others saying. Advocating for yourself, or having people with you to help you advocate, is always important, and especially so in an induction.

If you have a doula or other support people who will be with you during labor, it's great to plan when they'll be with you. Many people have a birth partner—a husband, wife, lover, coparent, best friend, sibling, parent—who'll be with them start to finish the entire time they're in the hospital. This can be helpful. Because inductions can be a very long process, if you have other support people, such as an older parent, you may want them to stay home and rest during the beginning of the induction and come in when you're closer to giving birth. With my clients, I join them *anytime* they'd like. For some that means they want me there from the beginning; for others they might check in frequently but get a medication like Cervidil overnight before having me join them the next day. Have a clear plan with your support people about when you want them with you, what you're expecting from them, and how you'll communicate.

It's common for people to get pain medication during an induction. In Yael's birth, avoiding an epidural was important. When she first heard she'd need to be induced, one of her concerns was a sense that an induction required an epidural. This is not the case. You can still make choices about what coping strategies you want to use, and, while inductions can be longer and more challenging because of all the monitors and IVs, an induction doesn't require you to have an epidural. For Wendy, she said that having a doula and a doctor who were supportive of her plan to not have pain medication was so important for her because an induction was already a compromise on so many of the things she'd wanted for her birth. Being able to hold on to this aspect of her experience helped her birth be a positive experience.

That said, if you're planning to have pain medication, communicate this with the staff from the beginning and make sure it's available as soon as you'd like it. For Nina, the epidural was a "game-changer" that made her birth experience so much better. For Erin, waiting for nearly twenty hours without an epidural is something she wouldn't do again. She said, "Looking back, I would have gotten the epidural earlier" and gotten more rest during the process. You can ask that interventions be timed around pain medication choices to ensure you're not in more pain than you are OK with.

People are often concerned that inductions result in more Cesareans, but the data isn't clear how big an impact, if any, induction has on the rate of vaginal delivery. Some studies even show lower rates of Cesareans with induction.[12] It's always a risk that your induction will not end in a vaginal birth. In my experience, one reason this might happen is because the baby is in a less optimal position when the induction begins and isn't able to navigate into a better position. In the days before an induction or even when you check into the hospital, ask your provider to confirm either with ultrasound or their hands what position your baby is in (and not just if they are head down, but which direction they're facing). If the baby is in a less optimal position (ideally they are facing toward your butt, not looking sideways or forward), you might consider trying the Miles circuit (an internet search will show you everything you need). This can help move the baby into a better position.

When I work with clients who're facing an induction, I remind them that this is their birth, and being induced doesn't have to make this any less a joyful, positive, respectful, compassionate, empowering experience of meeting their baby. What can you do to feel excited and hopeful or at least comfortable and heard? Whatever happens during your induction, remember that this is your body, your baby, your story to write.

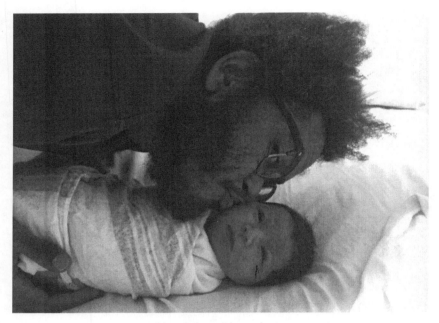

New father with newborn.

INDUCTION QUESTIONS

If your provider has scheduled an induction, or you're preparing for that possibility, asking some of these questions can give you a better sense of what to expect and what your preferences are.

WHY

- Why is an induction being recommended for me?
- Can you explain the risks of not being induced at this stage?
- Can you point me to some research on this?

WHERE

- Where will the induction take place?
- Am I in the hospital for the entire time?
- Do you do any elements of the induction in your office? Or send me home?

WHEN

- When are you recommending I be induced?
- What are my options in terms of when the induction happens?

WHAT

- What cervical ripening methods do you prefer to begin an induction with? Why?
- What induction medications do you have available? What do you routinely use?

WHO

- Who will be caring for me during the induction?
- Who will be there when I arrive?
- Who will administer the induction medications or place a cervical balloon if needed?
- If you work with a group practice, when do the doctors change shifts? Who is on next?
- Who can I bring with me for support?

HOW

- How can I avoid an induction?
- If necessary or desired, how can I best prepare for an induction?
- If desired, how can I refuse an induction that I do not believe I need?

HAVING A VAGINAL BIRTH AFTER A CESAREAN BIRTH

Jordan hoped for a vaginal birth but her water broke with her son still in a breech position. She headed to the hospital for a Cesarean. It was not what she'd wanted, but we worked to make it as positive an experience as possible. Afterward, I reminded her that this birth didn't have to dictate her future births. Three years later she mailed me a birth announcement. They'd moved across the country and had a successful vaginal birth after a Cesarean birth (VBAC) with her second baby. Along with a picture of her two boys together, she wrote on the back thanking me for being the first person to encourage her that she could have a VBAC in her future.

While not everyone is a great candidate for giving birth vaginally after a prior Cesarean, most people are. In 2013 the rate of people attempting a VBAC was 20 percent for pregnant people with one previous Cesarean birth and 7 percent for people with two or more previous Cesarean births. One study estimated that, if everyone who was a good candidate for a VBAC attempted one, the repeat Cesarean birthrate would drop from over 70 percent to about 25 percent,[1] and the vast majority of people who had a previous Cesarean birth are good candidates. There is an enormous difference between the number of people who are a good candidate for a VBAC and the number of people actually attempting a VBAC, so, like Jordan, I want to encourage you to consider a VBAC if it interests you.

Some people have heard that once you have a Cesarean birth, all future births will need to be via Cesarean. While that was the recommendation for a long time, it is not the case anymore. After giving birth via Cesarean, you usually have two options for subsequent births. The first option is to attempt "a trial of labor" after a Cesarean birth (TOLAC). A trial of labor is an obstetric term meaning you plan to go into labor and give birth vaginally. When a trial of labor is successful, it results in a vaginal birth (a VBAC), and when it is not successful, it results in an unplanned Cesarean birth. The second option is to have a planned repeat Cesarean delivery (PRCD). In what follows, I describe the benefits and the risks of planning a VBAC and the circumstances where that's a great option (as well as circumstances that make a repeat Cesarean birth safer). I then discuss strategies for a successful VBAC from selecting your provider and birth location, to preparing yourself for laboring and birth. Finally, I end with a brief discussion of preparing for the possibility that a trial of labor could end in another Cesarean birth.

THE BENEFITS AND RISKS OF PLANNING A VBAC

You may have a wide variety of reasons you're considering a vaginal birth or a repeat Cesarean birth—some of them might be a clinical assessment of the risks and benefits; others might be personal. For some, a prior Cesarean birth was part of a negative, upsetting, or even traumatizing birth experience, and planning for something *different* is important. For others, their prior Cesarean birth was a positive experience, and navigating a new birth requires considering the different benefits of staying with what worked last time or trying something new.

I hear from pregnant people who've had a Cesarean birth often about what they're weighing in their decision to attempt a VBAC or plan a repeat Cesarean birth. For some people, the desire to experience a vaginal birth is a strong motivating factor. They might also be hoping for a faster or easier recovery with a vaginal birth, or a shorter hospital stay and a faster return to their normal activity. For some, they're hoping for their baby to reap the benefits of being born vaginally, such as the benefits to their microbiome and gut flora (see chapter 14). Sometimes people are hoping for a vaginal birth because they have concerns about the safety of having too many Cesarean births and mounting risks. A repeat Cesarean birth appeals to some people because they worry about the physical and emotional challenges involved with trying for a vaginal delivery but ending up in another Cesarean birth. If they might end up in an operating room again, they'd rather not labor for hours. The ease of scheduling a Cesarean birth and being able to control which doctor is there for the birth are also appealing to some. Finally, they may have fears about the risks involved with attempting a vaginal birth and concerns about their baby.

Part of the challenge in navigating the risks and benefits of planning either to give birth vaginally or have a Cesarean birth is that the risks and benefits for the pregnant person and their unborn baby don't necessarily always align. Further, while the data isn't as clear as it could be, overall it suggests the safest mode of delivery is a VBAC. The second-safest option is a planned Cesarean birth, followed by a trial of labor ending in a Cesarean birth during labor.[2] This is tough because you cannot achieve that safest option—the VBAC—without risking having a trial of labor that ends in a Cesarean birth.

The biggest, and scariest, risk for people who've had a previous Cesarean birth is the possibility of a uterine rupture, an opening of the uterus. While a uterine rupture can occur in anyone, having a scar on your uterus from a previous surgery increases the risk. The rupture can be complete, or more commonly, partial. Both are dangerous and can result in significant bleeding, a need for blood transfusion, and fetal distress. Having a planned Cesarean birth does not entirely remove the risk of a uterine rupture but the rate is higher during a trial of labor. Unfortunately, many providers are so risk averse they won't support VBACs at all, even though it's the safest option for the vast majority of people. Some providers also attempt to measure the scar thickness to estimate the chances of a uterine rupture, but there's no evidence to suggest this is an accurate or useful index for assessing risk. Unfortunately, there is no reliable method for predicting uterine rupture in a person who has had a previous Cesarean birth.[3]

Thankfully, uterine rupture is very rare no matter how you give birth, especially if you have the most common type of incision from your Cesarean birth: a low transverse uterine incision (typically a four- to six-inch incision across the very bottom of your belly). For most people attempting a VBAC, there's about a 1 in 200 or less risk of a partial or complete uterine rupture and an even smaller chance that such a rupture would result in needing a hysterectomy (removal of the uterus) or significant fetal distress or fatality.[4] For most providers, this is an acceptable level of risk to support VBACs in a clinical setting where access to emergency services is readily available. If you're in a facility where they're able to perform an emergency Cesarean, the data suggests the benefits of a vaginal birth likely outweigh the risks.

Your provider should review your surgical records from your previous Cesarean birth(s) to verify what type of uterine incision was made. While you might have a low transverse scar on your belly, this doesn't necessarily mean that the incision made in your uterus matches. If you had another type of uterine incision made, such as a classical, T-, or J-shaped incision, this greatly increases the risk of uterine rupture when attempting a VBAC (studies show a

4–9 percent rupture rate). Also, having a previous uterine rupture is a big risk factor for another uterine rupture (6–32 percent recurrence rates, depending on the previous type of rupture).[5] While the overwhelmingly likelihood is still that your uterine scar wouldn't rupture, the risks are much higher, potentially greatly outweighing the benefits of a vaginal birth. Finally, having two or more Cesarean births increases the chances of a uterine rupture (but research suggests with each successful VBAC, the risk of rupture lowers).[6]

Another risk associated with a prior Cesarean birth is the risk of placenta attachment issues, regardless of how you give birth. Once you've had a Cesarean birth or a uterine scar from another surgery, there's an increased risk that the placenta, in subsequent pregnancies, will attach to the scar tissue.[7] This increases the risk for placenta previa (a placenta that partially or entirely covers your cervix) and placenta accreta (the placenta growing too deeply into the uterine wall). While we don't know exactly what causes placenta accreta, scarring after Cesarean birth greatly increases the risk. Further, the more Cesareans births you've had, the greater the risk for placenta previa and accreta. This is a good reason to consider a VBAC, especially if you're planning future pregnancies.

Like all births, both VBACs and Cesarean births have some risk of infection. It's possible to develop an infection during labor, often from vaginal exams or internal monitors, and it's also possible to develop a postpartum infection. With a planned Cesarean birth there's no risk of developing an infection during labor, but rates of postpartum infection after a VBAC are lower than after a planned Cesarean birth. The highest rate of infection occurs when a trial of labor results in a Cesarean delivery.[8]

Sometimes providers or pregnant people also suggest that avoiding vaginal tearing or pelvic trauma is a benefit to planning a repeat Cesarean birth. It's true that there will be no vaginal tearing if you don't attempt a vaginal birth; however, pregnancy itself can cause issues with your pelvis regardless of how you give birth. This is not a clinically compelling reason to opt for a Cesarean birth unless you've had previous vaginal trauma or surgeries that have greatly increased your risk of severe tearing. That said, avoiding vaginal tearing might be personally compelling, even if not clinically supported, and a Cesarean birth might be preferred in this case.

In weighing the pros and cons of a planned repeat Cesarean birth or a VBAC, your health and history also make a significant difference. A big part of assessing the risks and benefits of either birth option is weighing the specifics of what happened with your last birth(s) and how things are progressing with this pregnancy. For example, if you've already given birth vaginally at least once, you have an even higher likelihood of having a VBAC. That said, if your previous Cesarean birth happened for a reason that is considered a reoccurring indication, such as failure to progress, the chances of a successful VBAC are lower. Age can also be a factor in planning a VBAC or a Cesarean birth because younger people have higher success rates with VBACs; however, I've helped many people well into their forties have VBACs. Being pregnant with twins should not alone be a reason to discourage a VBAC, as the risks and benefits of a VBAC are similar to being pregnant with a single baby. Not going into labor by your estimated due date is also not a clinically supported contraindication for a VBAC.[9] If your provider will not support you staying pregnant past forty weeks gestation, this might be an indication that they are less supportive of VBACs.

Some providers will caution against attempting a VBAC if your baby is suspected to be large, but this alone doesn't necessarily require a scheduled repeat Cesarean birth. There's some data that uterine rupture might be more common with a larger baby,[10] but the obstetric guidelines for recommending a Cesarean birth for a suspected big baby are over 5,000 g (over eleven pounds) in pregnant people without diabetes and 4,500 g (nearly ten pounds) in pregnant people with diabetes.[11] In the vast majority of cases, fetal weights are estimated well below this, and, once born, the babies are actually in the normal range for weight.[12] Even with gestational diabetes, while the overall rate of VBAC is lower, this isn't a contraindication for VBAC. If your provider is suggesting you have a Cesarean birth because of the size of your baby or your diabetes, you should speak with them further about how large they believe the baby is and anything specific about your health or history that would make a trial of labor less safe. Further, I've worked with many people who were strongly cautioned to restrict carbs or calories in an effort to not have a large baby. The data does not support this for people who don't have diabetes. While eating healthy food is always recommended, dieting is not.

One tool your provider might use in conversations about the risks and benefits of a vaginal birth is called a VBAC calculator. There are several calculators available, each aimed at predicting the chances a pregnant person will have a VBAC based on demographics and clinical risk factors. These calculators often account for information such as age, height, weight, BMI, being African American or Hispanic, previous vaginal birth (especially a previous VBAC), and if your Cesarean birth was for what is called arrest of dilation (if your cervix stopped dilating during active labor) or arrest of descent (if after your cervix was fully dilated your baby did not move lower in the birth canal without pushing). Based on this information, the calculator produces a percentage prediction of how likely you are to have a vaginal birth.

Sometimes calculators are used to counsel a pregnant person about their options, helping them realize they have a good chance of achieving a VBAC and that a Cesarean delivery might not be their safest option. This is generally considered a helpful tool for informing pregnant people of the full range of their birth options. That said, I've also seen providers use a calculator to strongly discourage a VBAC. This is a less ideal use of the tool, because VBAC calculators heavily rely on demographic factors such race and body size, which are as much, or more, about provider bias, privilege, sizeism, and racism as they are about clinical factors.

Weight/BMI are used to predict the likelihood of a VBAC, but I do not find this data compelling. While there is clinically no specific limitation on BMI/weight that should be used in considering a trial of labor, some providers restrict access to VBACs based on BMI. If your provider won't support a VBAC over a certain BMI/weight, you may want a second opinion from another provider. If your provider is using a calculator to discourage you from attempting a VBAC, this might be an indication of how supportive they are. Discuss with them (or a new provider if you opt to switch) your commitment to a VBAC and their willingness to support you.

Finally, there are many circumstances where having a repeat planned Cesarean birth is clearly a better plan than a VBAC. As with any pregnancy, there are circumstances where a vaginal birth is not safe, such as placenta previa, or not recommended, such as a breech baby. Your decision to have a VBAC or a Cesarean birth should be made in conversation with your provider, based on your preferences, and informed by the best evidence available. This conversation can begin before you become pregnant, and should continue as more information about your pregnancy becomes available.

PREPARING FOR A VBAC

When clients come to me who'd like a VBAC, I tell them I think there are two key factors that will play a huge role in their births (and neither are found in the VBAC calculators). The first factor is desire and motivation to have a VBAC—you often need to really want it in order to get a VBAC. This is not to say that wanting it will make it happen; many people have wanted a VBAC and needed a Cesarean birth. Rather, in a clinical system that tends to favor repeat Cesarean births, your own motivation will be key in advocating for a VBAC. Having your partner, if you have one, also be supportive is incredibly valuable. The second factor is the provider you select, because not all providers support VBACs.

Even among the providers who support VBACs, some are far more supportive than others. Many providers will say they support VBACs, but in practice they rarely do, preferring to schedule a Cesarean birth. Additionally, having the support of a doula can be very valuable for those planning a VBAC.

When picking your provider, it's good to be aware of the impact that the location where you give birth might have on your options. The ACOG recommends you have a VBAC in a birth location where an emergency Cesarean is immediately available, never at home or in a hospital that doesn't have these emergency services.[13] That said, as I have mentioned before, some birth centers and home-birth midwives do support out-of-hospital VBACs. Beyond this, policies about epidurals or other pain medications, your mobility, drinking or eating, when a repeat Cesarean birth is planned if labor does not begin, induction of labor, pushing positions, and more might vary hugely between providers and birth locations and are worth investigating. Some hospitals, for example, have policies about when you must give birth by, require an epidural, or prohibit induction. These types of policies might have a large impact on your birth and your choices.

For Elana, this meant that she traveled to a hospital further from her home to be with a midwife who was incredibly supportive of her giving birth vaginally but worked in a place where an OB was available to perform surgery immediately. This felt like "the right balance of giving me every chance of giving birth the way I wanted but acknowledging the risks and feeling safe." One week before her due date, her water broke and labor began. She drove an hour to the hospital, had the support of her midwife through twelve hours of labor, took a couple of naps after she got an epidural, watched some TV, and gave birth to her son vaginally.

For Sharon, she found the immediate availability of a Cesarean concerning. She knew a VBAC was safer for her than another Cesarean birth, but, when she met with local VBAC-supportive doctors, she felt like they were all very biased in favor of Cesarean birth. She opted to give birth with a midwife at home because she felt this was her best chance of actually having a VBAC. Sharon went into labor at night while the rest of her family was sleeping. She stayed in bed trying to sleep as the contractions became closer together and stronger, woke her husband eventually to help when things got too intense to manage alone, and pushed her baby out into her midwife's hands in a pool of water in her Queens apartment.

Finally, for Rae, a recent client of mine, her successful VBAC came after an induction in the hospital. Her providers scheduled a repeat Cesarean birth for one week after her due date, but she hoped (and planned) to have a baby vaginally before then. A week of contractions that came and went got her to 4 cm, but the baby hadn't come. We checked into the hospital for her Cesarean birth with her having uncomfortable contractions every six to eight minutes. As they began getting her ready for surgery, Rae was able to talk with her provider about the option of delaying the scheduled Cesarean and trying a low dose of Pitocin instead. Her provider agreed and moved us into a labor room. Five hours later she was 7 cm, and they turned the Pitocin off. After less than an hour of pushing and only eight hours of total labor, she gave birth vaginally to her nine-pound daughter.

While the data says VBACs are most successful when labor is not induced, Rae's experience highlights the value of a provider offering options to avoid an unwanted repeat Cesarean birth. It is also a nice example of the importance of being motivated to have a VBAC, as Rae was able to advocate for the birth she wanted. Some providers will not do anything to induce or augment labor, like Pitocin or breaking the water, but the data says both are safe options and can help more people have VBACs.[14] This is an example of something that might differ between providers, even providers who support VBACs, and why I believe that one of the key factors in a successful VBAC is who you choose as your provider.

When you're laboring after a Cesarean birth, labor is essentially the same as labor might be without a prior Cesarean. A key difference I've found is how you might feel about laboring based on your prior experience. For some people, their Cesarean birth was a positive experience and planning a VBAC is not an emotionally difficult process. For others, they have tears running down their face when they tell me their Cesarean birth story. Planning a VBAC might be something you really want, and it might also be something you are scared to want too much in case another Cesarean birth ends up being recommended or required.

You might have regrets about decisions you made (or that were made for you), the support you received, or the ways you were treated during your last birth. You might be making very different plans this time and hoping for a very different experience, even if you have another Cesarean birth. You might be fearful that you'll have another Cesarean birth, and this might be especially difficult if the things that happened last time begin to repeat. For example, when I have a client who stopped dilating at 3 cm last time, they might be hugely relieved by an exam that says they are 5 cm. Another client who stayed at 6 cm for hours before a prior Cesarean birth might be distraught if two exams in a row are 6 cm. Navigating your previous experience and your feelings about it are often very much a part of the experience of a VBAC. The support of a partner, doula, friend, family member, therapist, or support group like the International Cesarean Awareness Network (ICAN) can be invaluable as you prepare to give birth again.

As important as it is to plan for the experience of a VBAC, it's valuable to also have a plan for a trial of labor that ends in a Cesarean birth. Talking with your provider about your preferences if a Cesarean birth is necessary can be an important part of planning for a positive birth experience. Preparing yourself emotionally is also valuable. For some people, a trial of labor that ends in a Cesarean birth might be a difficult experience, and it's important to give yourself space to mourn or be upset or heal however you need. You can be thrilled you are healthy and have a healthy baby, even while being upset that things didn't go differently. And, it's also OK to not have big feelings about how you give birth. Planning a VBAC and needing a Cesarean birth might be something you feel more neutral about.

For some people, it might be a healing experience to have a second Cesarean birth. Anita described her unplanned Cesarean after a trial of labor that way. With her first, she labored for many hours but never dilated beyond about 4 cm. Her baby became very distressed, and she had a Cesarean birth. Four years later she planned a VBAC, but labor took a familiar course. After hours of labor, her water broke and was very brown, meaning her baby had pooped inside. She was 4 cm when she arrived at the hospital, and the baby looked healthy on the moni-

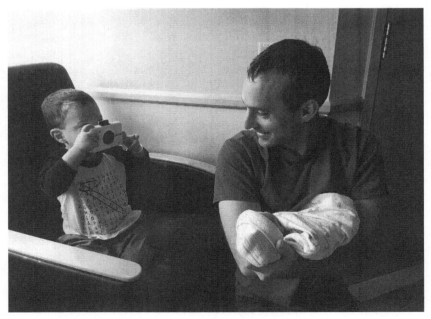

Big brother meeting his sibling for the first time.

tors. After a day of laboring, her cervix was still 4 cm open, the baby had begun to show signs of distress, and Anita had developed a fever (from infection likely). It was time for a Cesarean birth. This was both disappointing and familiar. She told me, "Needing a second c-section was actually a really healing experience in many ways." She explained: "I wanted a vaginal birth and I felt like if I'd done things differently the first time, I might have never needed a c-section." This time she worked with new doctors, at a different hospital, avoided an induction, and her water broke at home but, as she noted, "everything went the same. And that was actually helpful. It made me feel at peace with my first birth. It helped me know that I had birthed my babies the way they needed to be born."

Planning a VBAC and needing a Cesarean birth is not a failure. Nor is wanting a Cesarean birth and opting not to try for a VBAC. However you give birth, a vaginal birth or a Cesarean birth, planning for an experience that feels good for you and where you have support, encouragement, and your needs met can make this a positive experience.

FINDING A VBAC-SUPPORTIVE CARE PROVIDER

In most areas, both OBs and midwives support patients attempting a VBAC, and in many areas, you might have the options of birthing in a hospital or at home. Lots of providers might suggest they are VBAC supportive, but having policies and practices that actually support VBAC will significantly increase your odds of having a vaginal birth. Asking questions of potential providers early on can help you find a provider who will support you in the birth you want:

- Do you support patients who are planning a TOLAC/VBAC?
- Where do you practice? (Which hospital? At home?) Why do you feel this is a good birth location for having a VBAC?
- If you practice in a hospital, how supportive are the policies of the hospital toward people attempting a VBAC?
- How often have you worked with pregnant people who are attempting a TOLAC/VBAC? Do you have a sense of how often your patients who seek a VBAC give birth vaginally?
- Would you require me to have an epidural, or will you support an unmedicated birth if I prefer? If I would like an epidural, do you place any limitations on when I can have it?
- If signs of fetal distress are noted on the monitors during labor, will you attempt to resolve the distress and confirm the extent of the decelerations (by repositioning me, using an internal monitor, checking my pulse, etc.) before a Cesarean birth is called?
- If I'm not in labor, will you strip my membranes in the days prior to a repeat Cesarean birth to stimulate labor?

- Will you consider rupturing my membranes to see if labor will begin prior to a repeat Cesarean birth?
- If I am in labor, are you comfortable giving low-dose Pitocin if augmentation could be helpful in achieving a VBAC?
- If I am not in labor, would you consider giving me low-dose Pitocin to induce labor?
- At what point would you schedule a repeat Cesarean birth? At thirty-nine weeks? At forty weeks? At forty-one weeks? After forty-one weeks? Why?
- Do you place limits on the estimated fetal size when supporting clients in seeking a TOLAC/VBAC?
- Do you place limits on a client's weight when supporting a TOLAC/VBAC? Is there a maximum amount of weight I can gain before you would not support a TOLAC/VBAC?
- Will you support a TOLAC for patients who've had more than one previous Cesarean birth?
- Given my previous birth experience, do you believe that I'm a good candidate for a VBAC, and would you support me in that?
- Do you recommend I do anything to increase my chances of a having a VBAC (taking a class, hiring a doula, seeking out any type of complementary care like a chiropractor or a physical therapist)? Can you recommend anyone?
- Do the other providers whom you share on-call time with equally support VBAC, or do some of the providers in your practice have different policies or practices with VBAC?
- In the event that a repeat Cesarean birth becomes recommended or required, are you able to offer gentle Cesarean birth techniques including a clear drape to see the birth, and skin-to-skin contact with the baby in the operating room?
- Are the other providers whom you share on-call time with equally supportive of gentle Cesarean birth?

13

GIVING BIRTH TO TWINS/MULTIPLES

Finding out you're pregnant with twins or multiples might be incredibly exciting news, something you'd hoped for. It might also be overwhelmingly scary news or something you really hoped would not happen to you. Katherine described finding out she was pregnant with twins as an absolute shock. An ultrasound at six weeks appeared to show one baby, exciting news after trying to get pregnant for some time, but at an eight weeks visit with a local midwife everything changed. Katherine said, "It was an off the cuff decision to do a quick ultrasound in her office. She admitted she was not very experienced with ultrasounds and brought in a colleague to double check her work." The colleague confirmed: Katherine was pregnant with twins.

Katherine remembers leaving the office in a fog, stopping in a pizza shop, and calling her husband. The shock of finding out she was having twins lasted, she said: "I am not sure when that shock really wore off—not during the entire pregnancy and maybe not even for the first year of their lives!" She had conflicting feelings about the news. Other people remarked that she was lucky, but she felt "kind of angry that this totally improbable thing was happening to me."

Katherine is among the almost 3.5 percent of pregnant people in the US who give birth to twins every year. In 2016 there were just under 132,000 twins, about 3,800 triplets, more than 200 quadruplets, and 31 quintuplet or higher-order births in the US.[1] The number of multiple pregnancies in the US has increased in recent decades, with the rate of pregnant people giving birth to multiples currently about twice as high as it was in the 1970s. Fertility treatments have contributed to this increase in multiple pregnancies: both IVF (where an egg is fertilized outside the body and an embryo, or multiple embryos, are transferred into the body) and prescription fertility medications increase the odds of multiple pregnancies.

Another factor increasing multiple pregnancies is people giving birth later in life (twins are more likely when you are over thirty because you're more likely to release two or more eggs at a time). Additionally, some data suggest that both higher weight and height can contribute to the likelihood of having twins, as well as being African American. If you have given birth several times already, if you got pregnant while you're chest/breastfeeding, or if you have a family history of fraternal twins, these factors might also increase your odds of having twins.[2]

However you become pregnant and whatever you're feeling—happy, excited, lucky, overwhelmed, scared, angry—navigating a pregnancy with more than one baby is both the same as a single pregnancy in some ways and also totally different. In what follows, I briefly explain the differences between identical and fraternal twins/multiples (zygosity) and the significance of sharing a placenta and amniotic sac or having separate placentas and sacs (chorionicity). I then turn to the elevated risks in multiple pregnancies and what to expect during your prenatal care. Finally, I discuss both vaginal and Cesarean birth with multiples, and the decisions you can make about where you give birth, your provider, and your birth preferences.

TYPES OF TWIN/MULTIPLE PREGNANCIES: ZYGOSITY AND CHORIONICITY

Multiple pregnancies vary in number (twins, triplets, more), genetics (fraternal versus identical), and also in the number of placentas/amniotic sacs you have. The vast majority, 97 percent, of multiple births in the US are twins pregnancies,[3] so I've largely focused on twins pregnancies in what follows. As well, the vast majority of twins are fraternal (or dizygotic) with only about 3 percent of all twins being identical (monozygotic).[4]

Fraternal multiples result from two different fertilized eggs, and they have their own placenta and amniotic sac (dichorionic/diamniotic). Identical multiples result from the splitting of one fertilized egg. Identical twins can have two placentas and sacs (dichorionic/diamniotic), one placenta and sac (monochorionic/monoamniotic), or one placenta and two sacs (monochorionic/diamniotic), depending on the timing of the egg division.

Early on, your provider should be able to begin assessing the zygosity and chorionicity of your pregnancy with ultrasound. They may be able to identify

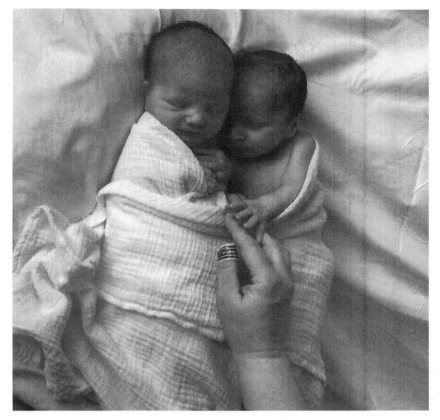

Fraternal twin newborn brothers.

two placentas (or one) but it's worth noting that they're not always correct. Two placentas can appear fused, looking like one (especially later in pregnancy), and more rarely, one placenta can have lobes that make it look like two on the ultrasound. Your provider can also determine if there's an intertwin membrane to determine how many amniotic sacs there are. Much like determining the number of placentas, it's possible to misidentify the intertwin membrane.

Especially if you've been undergoing fertility treatments, it's not uncommon to have ultrasounds very early, and multiples can be identified as early as four weeks. It's possible an early ultrasound will detect twins, but, by later ultrasounds, there will no longer be twins (called a "vanishing twin"). This type of early spontaneous reduction from a twin pregnancy to a singleton pregnancy occurs frequently (15–36 percent of the time).[5] For some people, this may be experienced as a significant loss and it's important to give yourself space to mourn that loss and process your potentially complicated feelings: the joy in the pregnancy you still have and the sadness of the birth loss. This may also not be something you experience as a loss, and your feelings on it may not feel complicated at all.

By the beginning of the second trimester, your provider can identify fetal sex. The most common type of twins are male-female (or boy-girl) twins, and they're all fraternal. All identical twins are same sex (both female or both male), but many fraternal twins are also the same sex, so this alone doesn't help in determining if they're identical.

This might sound confusing, and it is, even to experienced sonographers and doctors who specialize in multiple pregnancies. While it's *often* possible to determine with a great degree of certainty zygosity and chorionicity, it's not *always* possible. For example, some parents find out later (with DNA tests) that what they believed were fraternal twins are in fact identical. It's useful to do ultrasounds to assess chorionicity, even if it's not always correct, because knowing how connected or separated your twins are can help in monitoring and managing your pregnancy.

MONITORING AND MANAGING RISKS IN A TWINS/MULTIPLE PREGNANCY

Being pregnant with twins/multiples is considered higher risk, and this changes how you will be monitored and treated during pregnancy. It will also likely change your options for care providers, birth locations, and the likelihood of a Cesarean birth being recommended or required. While there are specific differences in risk based on the number of placentas and amniotic sacs, all multiple pregnancies carry a risk for growth restriction and preterm birth. With the exception of postdate pregnancy (going past forty-two weeks) and having a very large baby (two risks that aren't significant in multiple pregnancies), almost all other pregnancy risks are higher when you're pregnant with multiples.

Beyond the risks of preterm birth and growth restriction, there are other risks for twins that vary based on the type of twins. Sharing one placenta and one amniotic sac is riskier than each baby having their own placenta and sac. For example, monochorionic twins pregnancies can be complicated by disorders of the shared placenta where blood flow is unevenly distributed, favoring one fetus. This uneven flow can lead to anemia and growth restriction in one fetus. Monochorionic twins also have more congenital anomalies than dichorionic twins and singletons. Additionally, monoamniotic twins are at an increased risk for cord complications where their cords become entangled, potentially compromising placental blood flow.

These risks are accompanied by a lot of potential complications with your own health that increase when you're pregnant with multiples, regardless of their chorionicity or zygosity. For example, in all types of twin pregnancies, high blood pressure and preeclampsia are more common, as are cholestasis of pregnancy, iron deficiency anemia, and a severe form of morning sickness (hyperemesis gravidarum). People who are pregnant with multiples have more blood flow changes in their body than singleton pregnancies, making more work for your heart, which can cause complications for some people. And, there is an increased risk of Cesarean birth in multiple pregnancies.

Due to all of these increased risks, you should expect that your prenatal care might be different than it would be if you were pregnant with a singleton. In my experience, most providers monitor your health and the development of your babies more closely with frequent checks of your blood pressure and urine, frequent ultrasounds including routine growth scans, earlier and sometimes more checks of your glucose tolerance (to rule out gestational diabetes) and your blood work (to rule out anemia or low iron), and more prenatal visits overall during pregnancy. This additional monitoring might be really welcome and reassuring. Susan, for example, said, "I had a lot of ultrasounds—every two weeks. I loved having all of these extra chances to see that they were doing well."

One thing that may be monitored less is your weight gain. Where weight gain checks and commentary about controlling weight gain are very common in singleton pregnancies, and a source of stress for some people, you're more likely to find yourself being encouraged to gain weight if you're pregnant with twins or multiples.

The likelihood of bed rest (a prescription to stay in bed or otherwise limit activity) being recommended is higher with a twins/multiple pregnancy. What your provider means by bed rest can vary. They might mean: stopping or reducing the amount of work you're doing; avoiding sex; avoiding exercise, lifting, and anything strenuous; or they might mean actually resting in bed, sometimes even a hospital bed while being monitored, with a prohibition on almost all movement or activity. Bed rest might be recommended temporarily to help with a complication, or it could be recommended for the remainder of pregnancy. If your provider is recommending bed rest, you might want a second opinion. Studies show bed rest in twin pregnancies doesn't improve outcomes enough to warrant the risks associated with it.[6] Being immobilized and bedridden for long stretches of time can increase risks, such as the risk of dangerous blood clots, and it is generally not good for your emotional/psychological well-being.

Finally, given all of the monitoring in a twin pregnancy, your provider might have additional doctors as part of your care team. If you are seeing an MFM, they will do this themselves, but if you are seeing a midwife or non-MFM doctor, they will usually consult with an MFM. When you interview providers, gather this information so you're clear on who you'll be seeing prenatally (and during birth).

GIVING BIRTH TO TWINS/MULTIPLES

In many ways, giving birth to twins or multiples is the same as giving birth to a singleton. The labor process is the same with contractions causing the cervix to thin and open while the baby's head descends further into the birth canal. The signs and symptoms of labor can be very much the same, such as the passing of your mucus plug, contractions, feeling nauseous or throwing up, feeling shaky, having your water break (or be broken), bloody show, and rectal pressure. For many people, laboring with twins doesn't change any of these aspects of the labor process.

Similarly, having a Cesarean birth with twins (or multiples) is not significantly different than with a singleton. You'll still be in an operating room with anesthesia. Your provider will still aim to make a small, low, horizontal incision in both your abdominal wall and uterus to deliver your babies through. The policies in your hospital about Cesarean birth and the options for things like support in the operating room, seeing the birth, and skin-to-skin contact with your babies if they are healthy and stable should be the same.

One major difference is that twins almost always arrive earlier, often because your body goes into labor preterm. It's important to be aware of the signs of preterm labor, including:

- Any menstrual-like cramping that comes and goes or feels more constant
- A dull backache in your lower back
- Pressure in your pelvis
- More than four contractions in an hour
- Intestinal cramping with or without diarrhea
- Increased vaginal discharge, especially mucus or watery discharge leaking out of you

If you're experiencing any of these symptoms, it may be a sign that you are having contractions or that your cervix is beginning to open. You should contact your provider.

While it might be an option for you to give birth to twins/multiples in a birth location other than a hospital, it's very uncommon. There are some midwives who will support homebirth with twins, or even triplets, under specific circumstances (like staying pregnant until at least thirty-six or thirty-seven weeks with no health complications for yourself or your babies and having the first baby be head down, for example). Midwives who support out-of-hospital multiple births are rare, so you may have to travel to find someone if this is important to you. Further, the laws in your state (or the state where the midwife works) might make offering this service illegal (in which case you can expect that insurance will not cover it).

Years ago, a former client of mine rented a cabin in another state and paid cash for midwifery services in order to give birth to twins outside of a hospital. Another person I know hired local midwives for her second pregnancy, with triplets, and delivered all three in a tub in her living room. Both of them had great birth experiences and felt proud. That said, there are very significant risks associated with giving birth to multiples outside a hospital, greater than with a singleton pregnancy. Speak with potential midwives if you're considering a homebirth and create a solid transfer plan for preterm labor or complications your midwife can't treat at home.

Katherine had given birth to her first child with midwives and hoped to do so again. The news that she was expecting twins changed this: "Being pregnant with twins closed a lot of doors for me. It felt like it was shutting me out of my ideal birthing situation. The midwife I had picked was no longer an option, the birth center was out because twins are considered too high risk." She found a midwife who was open to caring for her, but had almost no experience (she'd been to two twins births). Katherine said, "I was trying to convince myself it might be ok to work with someone so inexperienced but it wasn't." She said, "Everything I read led me to decide that I needed to find an obstetrician to support me in this birth," so she began looking for a doctor. She wanted "someone who would let me give birth to twins how I wanted to, and that was elusive." After seven interviews, she settled on someone she felt was "as good as it gets."

Katherine moved on to finding a doula, interviewing someone recommended on a local twins group. She described that meeting, saying, "We told her about our first birth, the birth we were hoping to have this time, and the process we'd been through to find our obstetrician. She was concerned that the OB we'd picked was not a good match for our plans." The doula "knew every one of the doctors we'd met, all the hospital policies and procedures, the limitations in a twins birth, and recommended two other groups we hadn't yet considered (both at a hospital we had also not considered)." Katherine almost rejected the option of meeting more providers, feeling like she was making things too complicated, but ultimately she reached out to the doula's first choice and loved them.

Depending on where you are located, you may have a lot of options for providers, like Katherine did. Or there may be very few local options who have significant twins experience. Asking other local families with twins about their birth experience or seeking out local doulas with twins experience can be a helpful place to start gathering information about your options.

Describing her birth, an unmedicated vaginal birth of twin boys, Katherine said, "Some of what happened to me was sheer luck, and I get that, but some of it was not luck." She said it was worth finding a doula to help her advocate for the birth she wanted, and it was worth "meeting an insane number of care providers in order to find the people who would support me in birthing my way." Katherine acknowledged that as much as she feels lucky, she also feels "really proud" of herself for doing all the work, even when it felt like the odds were stacked against her.

While the estimated due date given to pregnant people is at the forty-week mark, it's rare for twins or multiples to gestate this long. Most providers adjust your due date to thirty-seven or thirty-eight weeks with twins (and often schedule an induction or Cesarean at that point or sooner if you haven't given birth). Being born preterm (before thirty-seven weeks) significantly increases the risk of one or more of your babies needing to spend time in the NICU for help with things like breathing and feeding. Given this, you may want to talk with your provider about when they'll recommend a routine induction or Cesarean birth. Among my clients, this has varied from as early as thirty-five weeks to as late as thirty-nine or forty weeks, without complications or reasons for earlier delivery. With such a range of recommendations, and knowing the increased risks associated with preterm birth, this is something you may want to consider when picking a provider.

Additionally, Cesarean births are the most common method of delivery for twins and happen more than 60 percent of the time.[7] This is partially because it is more common for the lowest baby (baby A) to be breech. It's also partially due to provider preference for Cesarean births, sometimes because they lack training and experience with multiple vaginal births. The current rate of Cesarean births for multiple pregnancies is higher than it needs to be. Studies have shown that increasing the number of twins born vaginally would be safer, improve outcomes, and avoid unnecessary risks associated with surgical birth.[8] Given this, unless you have a strong preference for a Cesarean birth, it's important to find a provider that routinely supports vaginal births and is comfortable and confident in helping you.

For a vaginal birth with twins in the hospital, there will typically be some differences in how your labor and birth are supported. For example, most providers will require continuous fetal monitoring during labor and might recommend using one internal fetal monitor and one external monitor to make sure they accurately track both heartbeats. It's also common for providers or hospital policy to require having an epidural during labor with twins, which might be something you're comfortable with or it might be something you're hoping to avoid.

Susan picked high-risk OBs at a local hospital where vaginal twins were common, but she knew up front that they required an epidural during labor. While she agreed to this, she did insist on delaying it. She said, "I know the nurses thought I was crazy, but it was my choice, so I waited until 6cm." Prior to getting the epidural, she was imagining "a Hawaiian hot spring" during the contractions. The water was, "really warm, almost too hot," and she focused on breathing through that imagined heat to cope with the contractions.

Having the epidural in place was helpful later when her second baby was born. After her son was born, her daughter was still "laying sideways across my uterus and up high, floating in her amniotic sac." Susan's OB wasn't confident about delivering her second baby vaginally, with limited experience, but was assisted by a more experienced MFM. The MFM tried to talk her OB through the delivery but ultimately took over when her OB became too nervous. Susan had what's called a breech extraction—where a doctor reaches inside your uterus and brings the baby down in a breech position to be delivered. The MFM described what he was doing: "Find a limb and grab on to it. Then you pull the baby down towards you and break the water." The doctor "pulled her left leg out, then her right leg, supported her as her butt came out, then her shoulders." Susan said, "I can remember the feeling of him cork screwing her back and forth to deliver her head last." With four minutes between births, both of her babies were born in what she described as "exactly the birth I wanted. My dream birth."

Another requirement for most multiple births is being in an operating room, even for a vaginal birth. Your providers may have you push in a labor room but move to an operating room shortly before birth, in case your second baby requires a Cesarean birth. While it's uncommon to have one baby born vaginally and one born via Cesarean, especially if your providers are experienced with breech extraction, being prepared to rapidly change course is safer.

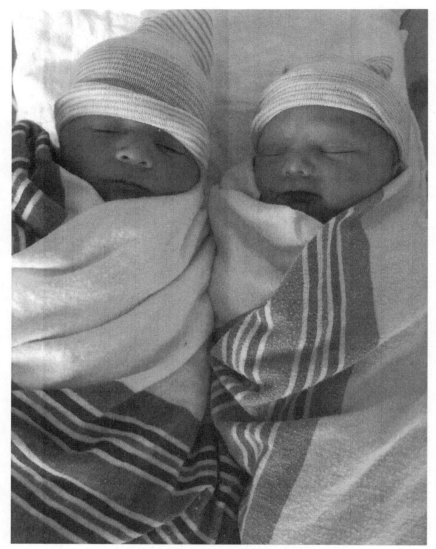

Newborn twins swaddled in a hospital bassinet together.

When I helped Shana give birth to her sons, her labor was induced at thirty-seven weeks. She got an epidural, as required, and her labor progressed smoothly. She was moved into an operating room with her first son very near to being born. Her team of doctors included three of the most experienced MFMs in NYC who deliver vaginal multiples. In more than six hundred vaginal twins births, they'd only once converted to a Cesarean birth for the second baby.

After Shana's first son was born, her second baby remained high up and head down. Her doctors wanted to turn him to deliver feet first, but he was hard to get ahold of. Getting him low enough to break the amniotic sac proved more difficult than expected. With one doctor pressing on her baby through her belly, another doctor was able to break the water, but his cord came out with the water and the baby was now transverse across Shana's uterus. Compounding the problem, her uterus was contracting powerfully around him, making it harder to turn him. Her doctors gave her medication (terbutaline) to relax her uterus, but it didn't help. They managed to get one of her son's feet out of her body, but, unfortunately, the baby was now presenting with both his head and feet down, crowding the space and making it impossible to bring him out feetfirst. After nine chaotic minutes of trying to deliver him vaginally, his heart rate was dropping and they converted to a Cesarean birth. While Shana's birth was rare, the decision to have her already in an operating room proved critical.

It's also common to have an extra-large medical team present when you give birth to twins/multiples (vaginal or a Cesarean birth). During labor you might have a normal-sized team of support people—primarily interacting with just one nurse, whomever you brought for support, and your doctor/midwife. When you're ready to give birth, however, your team might become much larger. It's common to have an anesthesiologist or two in the room, several doctors, at least one nurse per baby, one nurse for you, a team of pediatricians for each baby, and often in a teaching hospital, some residents, medical students, or student nurses as well. As Susan said: "With two babies, you get two of everything. I had two doctors, two teams of pediatricians, and two sets of nurses, as well an anesthesiologist, my doula, and my husband. Full house!" For Shana's birth, a group of students were there to see their first vaginal birth of twins, crowding the room with more than twenty people including her husband and me.

After your babies are born, depending on their age and health, they may need to spend some time in a NICU or they might be able to stay with you from the beginning. There can be more challenges associated with chest/breastfeeding twins or multiples, and working with an experienced lactation consultant from the beginning might be very helpful if nursing is important to you. You may also want to secure extra help postpartum before you bring your babies home, as there's a lot of work involved in caring for multiple newborns, especially while you recover from birth.

FINDING A SUPPORTIVE TWINS/MULTIPLES CARE PROVIDER

Many providers who care for people pregnant with twins or multiples only provide support for Cesarean birth. Others have rules about anesthesia or induction that aren't made readily available in advance. Asking questions when you interview a provider can help ensure you understand what to expect and that you've found someone who is a good match to your preferences.

- How many times have you delivered twins/multiples? What percentage were delivered vaginally? Is this the same for all the doctors/midwives in your practice?
- What do you require in order to attempt a vaginal delivery? What position do the babies need to be in? What size difference between baby A and B are you comfortable with for a vaginal twins birth? Is this the same for all the doctors/midwives in your practice?
- Do you offer breech extraction for baby B after the delivery of baby A? Is this the same for all the doctors in your practice?
- If breech extraction is not something you offer, is there an option to have an additional doctor present who does offer breech extraction?
- How often have you delivered baby A vaginally and then delivered baby B via a Cesarean birth? Is this the same for all the doctors in your practice?

- If I am planning a vaginal birth, what should I expect during labor?
  - Will a hep lock be required?
  - Will IV fluids be required?
  - Will intermittent fetal monitoring be available, or do I need to have continuous monitoring?
  - Do you routinely use internal fetal monitoring with twins?
  - How early in labor do you recommend breaking the water for internal monitoring?
  - Can I labor outside of the bed?
  - Will an epidural be required, or can I labor without pain medication if I prefer?
  - Will I need to deliver in an operating room?
  - Who can be with me in the operating room during a vaginal birth?
  - Does this vary between the doctors in your practice?
- Barring complications, at what point will you recommend an induction of labor?
- If I am induced, will you be the doctor with me for the delivery?
- If a Cesarean delivery is recommended or requested, do you offer gentle or family-centered Cesarean birth options? Will you perform the Cesarean yourself?

14

CESAREAN BIRTH

Grace made a hair appointment for the day before her scheduled Cesarean birth. She knew it might be a while before she could get it done again and hoped her hair would look good in her birth photos. As she sat in the salon chair, the stylist asked when she was due. This had come to feel like a loaded question for Grace. If she answered honestly, giving the stranger the date of her scheduled birth, this led to more invasive and judgmental questions and concerns about why she was having a Cesarean birth. She hated defending herself—proving to strangers that her Cesarean birth was necessary or justified. But, if she just gave her estimated due date and no other info, she was often subjected to lots of conjecture about when the baby might arrive: "First time moms are always late" and "You better be ready because you look like you're about to blow!" Even more troubling, there were follow-up questions and comments about her imagined plans: "Are you going to try natural?" or "Get the drugs, you're going to want them!"

Grace wasn't conflicted about her plans, or ashamed of having a Cesarean birth, but she was frustrated with comments, questions, and judgments. When her stylist asked when she was due, she chose honesty, replying that the baby would be born the next morning. After Grace clarified that she was having a Cesarean birth, the stylist inquired why. Grace calmly explained that asking about a medical diagnosis felt impolite and unnecessary. Her hair appointment was supposed to be about feeling good and taking care of herself. Grace asked if they could talk about something else. The stylist awkwardly mumbled apologies and turned on the blow dryer, silencing further conversation.

CHAPTER 14

The next morning in Grace's apartment, I took pictures as she finished getting ready. She was full of energy, even with the sun not up yet. Her hair looked great. She was nervous, and complained a bit about being thirsty and hungry (eight hours of presurgery fasting will do that), but mostly it was her optimism and enthusiasm I remember. She'd be meeting her baby in a few hours, and she'd be celebrating this day—her daughter's birthday—for the rest of her life. She walked into the hospital with a huge smile, welcomed her IV and monitors, and hugged her doctor when he arrived. In recovery, she was numb at first and later sore, but even with EKG leads taped to her chest, Grace was focused on stroking and kissing her daughter. Her wife stood next to her, eyes red from crying. It was, without question, one of the best days of their lives.

Cesarean births are one of the most common surgical procedures done in the US today. They're more common than removing tonsils or the appendix—so common that many hospitals have expanded their operating rooms and staff to accommodate them. In the 1970s, the Cesarean birthrate in the US was about 5 percent. Today, about 32 percent of births are surgical.[1] Some doctors have suggested this rise in Cesarean birth reflects an older population of pregnant people and more high-risk pregnancies, which is partially true, but the increase in Cesareans births is happening across all age groups and all types of pregnancies.[2] Cesarean birthrates vary hugely between individual providers, hospitals, and states, but everywhere in this country Cesarean births are common. Even if you're not planning for a Cesarean birth, preparing for the possibility is important for anyone who is pregnant.

People feel very differently about Cesarean births—some people will do almost anything to avoid it, others prefer it—and I honor all of the feelings people have about Cesarean births in this chapter. In what follows, I describe the experience of having a Cesarean birth to give you a sense of what's typical and to be expected. I also distinguish between four loose categories: elective, required, recommended, and emergency Cesarean births. I describe the reasons people have Cesarean births and evidence-based recommendations for reducing the Cesarean rate. I then detail the risks of Cesarean birth, and finally, I conclude with ways to advocate for the most positive, gentle Cesarean birth. Even while talking about the risks of Cesarean births and evidence-based recommendations for reducing the Cesarean rate, I also want to be really clear that Cesarean births are neither "failed" births, nor "less than" other births. I want to honor people, like Grace, who give birth surgically—for whatever reasons. It's a brave act of love to have surgery to bring your baby into the world.

WHAT ARE CESAREAN BIRTHS?

It's unclear when the first Cesarean was actually performed or how it got the name. There's evidence of Cesarean births in stories and artwork across cultures and throughout history. Julius Caesar is often cited as the namesake for Cesareans, but it seems likely this isn't the case.

A Cesarean birth is the birth of a baby, or babies, through an incision made in the abdominal wall and uterus. Cesareans are performed in operating rooms with a team of doctors (obstetricians, anesthesiologists, pediatricians) and nurses. Usually, you're brought into the operating room and given spinal anesthesia, so you're awake and alert. Doctors and nurses prepare the operating room and your body for surgery by arranging you on the operating table, placing sterile coverings on much of your body, and cleaning your skin.

After they've finished preparing, they typically allow you to have one or two support people brought in to the OR to be with you. Your support people are typically seated next to you, very close to your head. There's a drape or curtain stretched across your chest that functions to create a sterile field for the doctors to work, but it also blocks your view, and the view of your support people, so watching the birth is not typically an option (although this is increasingly negotiable if seeing the moment of birth is desirable to you).

During a Cesarean birth, you're flat on your back on an operating room table, which can be uncomfortable. One of your arms is usually strapped down to secure an IV for fluids and medications. Antibiotics are typically administered through the IV to prevent infection, and you may be given additional medications for pain, nausea, or other concerns specific to your health. Usually, your other arm is free to hold hands with your support person and touch your baby.

While you're not typically able to see the surgery, you and your support people will be in an operating room, so the tools, sounds, and smells of surgery are present. This can be scary. It's common for doctors to speak with each other about the surgery, or teach a student, so wearing headphones, talking to your support person, or asking to minimize talk about the procedure can help if you might be stressed by these sounds. Stephanie "banned any talk about what was going on below the curtain," which her doctors respected, so there was "a small army of strangers who were discussing Halloween plans" during her birth. She described her birth, saying:

> My husband, his blue eyes bright below the blue surgical cap, came into the room after they had prepared me for the surgery. He pulled out his phone to show me pictures of Lulu, our puppy. This was an approved distraction strategy. A few

photos in, I felt the tiniest, dull tug toward my chest. "Oh, he's coming," I said matter-of-factly. Not only had the surgery started, I just realized—it was about to be over. Not nearly as bad as I had thought it might be. Not even remotely as scary as I imagined.

With talk of the surgery banned and her husband showing her pictures of their puppy, Stephanie minimized her anxiety and fears about giving birth in an operating room. She had a birth that was "the opposite of what I had hoped for and imagined but still really positive all the same."

Stephanie's description of feeling a "dull tug" during her birth is not uncommon, but individual experiences vary. The anesthesia should block all sensations of pain, but you'll still feel pressure and the sensation of touch and movement. For a Cesarean birth, your doctor typically makes as small an incision possible, usually four to six inches horizontally, through the skin at the base of your belly above your pubic bone. The abdominal muscles are not cut; instead, they are pulled apart to provide access to your uterus, where a second incision is made to deliver the baby. In rare cases, usually emergencies, an incision is made laterally (from navel to pubic bone), but this isn't preferred as it complicates future pregnancies and makes VBACs less safe.

You shouldn't feel the incision itself at all, but following the incision, you'll likely feel varied amounts of pressure as the baby is born. For some people, this pressure can be intense and feel like someone is pressing on you forcefully or even, as Rehana said, "like someone was sitting on my belly." Others feel this as a sensation of having their body pushed or moved around or even, accurately, a feeling of "something being pulled out of me." Sam described her Cesarean birth as painless and said her scar was hardly noticeable. Her biggest memory was of shivering during the birth and then feeling pain as she recovered.

The entire experience typically takes just over an hour. Afterward, you're brought into a recovery room to continue being monitored. There's some preparation before the surgery, as noted above, but once the surgery is started, the baby is born within minutes. The placenta is removed quickly afterward. The majority of the time is spent on repair of the incision made in your uterus, and repair of the skin on your abdomen. Thankfully, having your baby born quickly tends to provide a wonderful distraction to any stress or anxiety you may be feeling. Hearing their cries, having the staff tell you your baby is doing well, and getting to see and hold your baby are usually moments of great relief and joy.

If your baby is born in a planned Cesarean birth, it may be possible to have the baby skin to skin quickly. More typically, babies are brought to pediatricians to be examined before they're wrapped and brought to your support person to hold. You can talk to and kiss your baby, and with your free hand you can help hold and touch your baby. You may be able to have your baby on your chest in the OR or in recovery, and you should be able to begin feeding if you'd like. Check with your hospital about what support is available in recovery and what help you may need with feeding or caring for yourself and your baby in the hours after birth.

ELECTIVE, REQUIRED, RECOMMENDED, AND EMERGENCY CESAREAN BIRTH

As a doula, I've worked with lots of people who've had Cesarean births for a wide variety of reasons, and while the vast majority of them were clearly the safest path forward, only a few of those births were true emergencies. The word "emergency" is used a lot to describe all sorts of unplanned Cesarean births, but actual emergencies are not common. Our language about Cesarean births feels too simplified and binary: necessary versus unnecessary, planned versus unplanned, scheduled versus emergency. There's no language in between to articulate the varied reasons why Cesarean birthrates top 50 percent in many US hospitals.

Part of the reason I think we lack good language to talk about Cesareans is because people have complicated feelings. For many people, avoiding ending up in an OR is a large part of their birth plan and weighs heavily on their decisions. For others, a Cesarean birth is preferable and desirable. There's no right or wrong way to give birth to our babies, yet people regularly report they experience judgment and stigma about their Cesarean birth. When I spoke with Daisy about her birth, she highlighted the shame many people assumed she felt:

> After my birth, I remember a lot of people around me trying to comfort me, saying things like "C-sections are ok." There was a lot of stigma and an assumption that I needed help processing the experience. People seemed apologetic. Many people I know had C-sections by choice, and while I would not have chosen this, this was the birth that my baby needed. Knowing her now, it does not surprise me at all that she picked a spot and stayed there. I have come to a place of really accepting that and feeling so confident that this was the right thing for my body and my baby. I did not have a Cesarean because it was the easiest thing to do or because it was convenient. I did it because it was what I had to do, and I do not regret that. I think there is often so much shaming about how we each give birth. In the end I felt really proud of how I gave birth.

In this context of stigma and people seeming apologetic about Daisy's birth, framing Cesareans as emergencies can feel compelling because it communicates that this was a "necessary" and, therefore, a good or acceptable reason to give birth surgically. If Cesarean births are framed as unfortunate, then having an "unnecessary" Cesarean means you were duped by an overly clinical system or uninformed and unthoughtful in your decision-making.

I wholly reject these hierarchies and judgments about how we give birth. In what follows, I use the term "elective" to describe births where surgery was requested by a pregnant person as their preferred method of delivery. I use the term "required" to refer to a prenatal diagnosis that's incompatible with vaginal delivery or not allowed in the location where you're giving birth. I use the term "recommended" to describe a Cesarean birth that happens during the course of pregnancy or labor at the recommendation of a provider but is neither an emergency, nor required (but isn't elective because there's a clinical indication for the recommendation). Finally, I reserve the term "emergency" for true emergencies where stat Cesareans are performed as a lifesaving surgery. I use this language—of elective, required, recommended, and emergency Cesarean

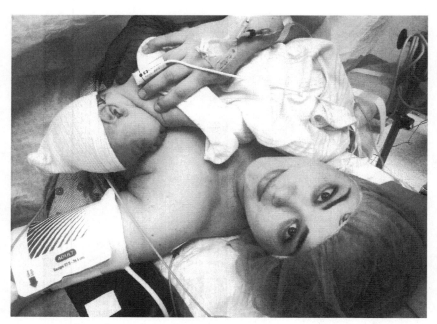

Newborn skin to skin in the operating room during a Cesarean birth.

births—to help you think about choice, consent, and control as you navigate your own pregnancy and birth.

REASONS YOU MAY WANT OR NEED A CESAREAN BIRTH

Within these categories of Cesarean births (elective, required, recommended, and emergency) there are differences in the ability to plan for or schedule. Elective Cesarean births are almost always planned in advance (although, it's also possible to change your mind during your labor and request a Cesarean birth), and emergency Cesareans are not planned for. Often, a Cesarean is required or recommended based on a prenatal diagnosis, and therefore able to be planned or scheduled ahead of time; others become recommended during the course of labor, and therefore are unscheduled.

Although elective Cesarean births are often cited as a reason why Cesarean rates in this country have increased dramatically in the last few decades, the data doesn't support this. Only a small percentage of Cesarean births, 1–3 percent, are classified as elective.[3] The reasons people elect to have a Cesarean are often trivialized with phrases like "too posh to push," and it's common for people to find themselves repeatedly being asked to defend this preference. I've worked with clients who wanted a Cesarean birth because they preferred the known and controllable elements of a scheduled surgery to the unpredictability of labor. Some of my clients have survived sexual abuse or assault and couldn't tolerate a vaginal delivery (although other survivors prefer a vaginal birth). I've worked with clients whose anxiety about a vaginal delivery was difficult to manage, and a scheduled Cesarean was calming and helped them have a better pregnancy. I've also worked with clients who had major vaginal trauma during a previous birth, or had friends/family who'd experienced serious complications, and preferred a Cesarean birth.

Whatever your reasons, if you'd prefer to have a Cesarean birth, this is absolutely a choice you can make. You'll want to work with a doctor, as midwives cannot perform Cesareans, and you'll want to speak with your doctor ahead of time to make sure they're supportive of your preference. Some providers will require that you first try for a vaginal delivery if there's no medical reason why it's unsafe. This policy may not be a good match for you if you'd prefer to schedule a Cesarean birth. Find a provider who's clear and confident about their support of your choice and respects your plan without trying to change it. Additionally, it's good to check your insurance coverage for elective surgery to make sure that your birth will be paid for.

Beyond elective Cesareans, many Cesarean births are also planned in advance because of a prenatal diagnosis that prompts this recommendation or requirement. Reasons you might have a Cesarean birth recommended or required prenatally include:

- A placenta that's too close to or covering your cervix, called **placenta previa**, makes cervical dilation dangerous and a Cesarean birth required. In some cases, when this is diagnosed very early in pregnancy, the growth of the uterus pulls the placenta way from the cervix, resolving the problem and making vaginal birth safe. In the third trimester, about 1 in 200 pregnant people have placenta previa.[4]
- Abnormalities in the baby's umbilical cord can also make a vaginal delivery dangerous. Normally the umbilical cord inserts into the middle of the developing placenta, but sometimes it is near the edge of the placenta (called a "marginal cord insertion"). Sometimes it doesn't insert into the placenta directly and the umbilical vessels run through the amniotic sac or membranes instead, called a **velamentous cord insertion (VCI)**. This happens in about 1 percent of singleton births but is more common with some types of twins, and it's also more common when there is a placenta previa.[5] When you have VCI, the vessels are not protected by the Wharton's jelly of the umbilical cord and are exposed and vulnerable. The most concerning form of a VCI is called a **vasa previa**, where those exposed vessels cross over or are near the cervix, because the water breaking can cause those vessels to rupture. Vasa previa occurs rarely, about 1 in every 2,500 births,[6] and is always considered cause for a required Cesarean birth. Some providers will also recommend a Cesarean if a VCI is diagnosed, but others will not. A marginal cord insertion is typically only cause for more monitoring during pregnancy and labor but not for a Cesarean birth.
- A Cesarean will also be required for any fetal or parental health concerns that make a vaginal birth unsafe. A fetal diagnosis, such as severe hydrocephalus, or "water on the brain," makes delivering via a Cesarean safer for the baby. A pregnant person with a uterine fibroid blocking the cervix, for example, will also require a Cesarean birth.
- A **breech** baby, one that's not head down in the birth canal, occurs about 3–4 percent of the time[7] and can prompt a recommended Cesarean birth. There are several types of breech presentation: a "complete breech" where the baby is butt down with both legs bent at the knees so the feet are down, a "frank breech" where the butt is down but both legs are

extended upward with the feet near the head, an "incomplete breech" where the butt is down but one leg is bent at the knee and the other leg is extended, and a "footling breech" where one or both feet are below the baby's butt and will deliver first. There are also two types of fetal presentation that may require a Cesarean: a "transverse lie" where the baby is lying sideways inside the uterus; and "an oblique lie," where the baby has their head on your hip and their body diagonal inside the uterus. In both cases, the baby can't be born vaginally unless it moves (or is moved by a provider). There are some providers and birth locations where a vaginal birth of some types of breech babies is possible, but most providers in the US recommend a Cesarean for a breech.

- A previous Cesarean birth used to mean all future births were required to be Cesarean births, but now most people who've given birth via a Cesarean are considered good candidates for a future vaginal delivery. There are also some previous uterine surgeries that may prompt your doctor to recommend or require a Cesarean delivery.

- Twins or multiples can be born vaginally, and often are, but there are more possible complications with multiples that can prompt a prenatal recommendation or requirement of a Cesarean birth. About 40 percent of twins are both head down, but, in the remaining 60 percent, at least one baby is in a breech position.[8] Some providers will support the vaginal birth of a breech second twin, as long as the first baby is head down. Others recommend a Cesarean for both babies. With triplets, there is even less likelihood of all three babies being head down. Studies suggest that, overall, routinely planning Cesarean births for twins and triplets is not safer than vaginal birth.

- **Macrosomia**, a suspected big baby, can prompt a recommended Cesarean birth. While there are some increased risks associated with especially large babies, this is not necessarily a good reason to consider a Cesarean birth. The American College of Obstetrician and Gynecologists (ACOG) doesn't recommend a scheduled Cesarean unless your baby is predicted to be over 5,000 grams (eleven pounds), which is substantially larger than the size of many babies I have seen OBs recommend a Cesarean birth for. Additionally, size estimates are frequently wrong, greatly overestimating the size of the baby. If you are concerned about an unnecessary Cesarean birth and your baby is measuring large, you may want to talk in greater detail with your provider about the risks associated with birthing larger babies, the data on when a Cesarean is recommended (and when it is not), and your preferences for your birth.

- Body size, or obesity, is also a common reason providers recommend a Cesarean birth. There is good reason to question this recommendation as Cesarean births carry more risks, especially for larger people.[9] What constitutes too big for a provider to support a vaginal birth varies, and some providers do not use body size as a criterion for mode of birth. There's no guideline for doctors on this recommendation.

Any health concerns or diagnoses may result in a recommended or required Cesarean birth, which can be planned or scheduled. Additionally, recommended, required, and emergency Cesareans can happen for a wide variety of unplanned reasons including:

- A **placental abruption**, where the placenta prematurely separates from the uterus. This happens in less than 1 percent of pregnancies and can be either a total or a partial separation.[10] When a placental abruption is suspected (a diagnosis can only be made after the birth; before that, it's just a suspicion based on symptoms), it can result in bed rest if the baby is stable, but when there's fetal distress or excessive bleeding, a Cesarean birth is necessary, often an emergency Cesarean.
- A **cord prolapse** is a rare complication where the cord comes out of the uterus before the baby after the water has broken. This occurs far less than 1 percent of the time (under 1 in 500 births) and is more common with breech babies.[11]
- Concerns for the well-being of the baby during the course of labor or before, usually diagnosed from an abnormal heart-rate pattern suggesting the baby is distressed, can prompt a Cesarean birth. Sometimes a concerning pattern emerges and prompts a recommendation to act before it becomes worse, and other times fetal distress can present as a prolonged deceleration in the baby's heart rate and prompt an emergency Cesarean. Fetal heart rates are classified into three types: category 1, 2, and 3. Category 1 tracings are a clearly healthy baby, and category 3 tracings are a clearly distressed baby. Category 2 is the more challenging category with lots of room for a clinician to interpret health or distress. In an effort to reduce the number of Cesareans, much attention is being paid to category 2 tracings and how fetal distress is diagnosed.
- Occasionally, a severe health concern such as preeclampsia, for example, is treated by delivering the baby. A vaginal delivery is often an option, but a Cesarean may be offered or required depending on the symptoms.

- During the course of labor, various factors can cause labor to progress slowly or a baby to not descend into the pelvis well. This can variously be called **labor dystocia** or obstructed labor, "failure to progress," or **cephalopelvic disproportion** (CPD) (meaning the baby is too large for the pelvis). It's often hard to assess how necessary these types of Cesareans are, and many people find themselves questioning whether more patience, different positioning, or alternative strategies could have resulted in a vaginal birth.

Many of the above reasons—such as a placenta previa, a vasa previa, a complete placental abruption, a true CPD, or a cord prolapse, among others—are medically indicated reasons to have a Cesarean birth. In those cases, all the data tells us with great certainty that a Cesarean birth is the safest (or only safe) way to give birth. The benefit of a Cesarean birth in these scenarios is overwhelming and profound, and no one would consider advocating otherwise.

Yet, the shift from a 5 percent Cesarean birthrate in the 1970s to one-third of births happening via Cesarean has caused concern about the overuse of surgical interventions. If you'd prefer a Cesarean birth, this is not a concern for you, but if your general preference is to avoid a Cesarean birth, then understanding how to navigate your options to avoid unnecessary intervention is important. Most Cesarean births are performed at the recommendation of a provider, so changes in how doctors perceive risk and what prompts intervention likely accounts for much of the rise in Cesareans. Health care policy makers and doctors disagree about exactly what percent of births should require a Cesarean birth—it's somewhere in the 10–20 percent range[12]—but nearly everyone agrees the rapid increase in Cesarean births in this country is not necessary or ideal.

If you're a pregnant person who'd prefer to avoid a Cesarean birth, it can be challenging to navigate situations where a Cesarean is recommended but not required. More than half of Cesarean births today happen for one of two reasons: fetal distress and failure to progress. While many Cesarean births are necessary, both of these reasons for a Cesarean birth have lots of room for individual provider interpretation of what constitutes distress, too little progress, or too much time spent in labor. Talking to your provider in advance can help you avoid a situation where you feel pushed toward an intervention you didn't want and aren't sure is necessary.

As I mentioned in chapter 8, ACOG and SMFM (the Society for Maternal-Fetal Medicine) released a statement in 2014 on safely preventing Cesarean births. Among their recommendations was a call to rethink how labor should progress, citing studies that confirm more time for labor to progress results in more people having vaginal births.[13] In your own search for a provider, if avoiding a Cesarean is something you'd prefer, you might ask specifically about their approach to managing longer labors and how tolerant they are of slower progress. During the course of labor, you might also check with your birth team if you're concerned about patience or too strict a timetable. Talk through your concerns, try to adjust expectations, and seek reassurance that you and your baby are doing well even if progress is not happening quickly.

Another recommendation made by the ACOG and SMFM is a reevaluation of what constitutes an abnormal fetal heart tracing and when action is required. Having too strict a sense of what a happy baby (or a distressed baby) might look like has caused more interventions than necessary. Altering how doctors interpret what warrants concern can increase the number of vaginal births without reducing health or safety. As noted above, fetal heart-rate tracings are divided into three categories, and more careful interpreting of category 2 tracings can decrease the number of Cesareans. Speaking to your provider in advance about their Cesarean rate and how they work to avoid unnecessary intervention is valuable.

An additional recommendation made by the ACOG and SMFM for avoiding Cesarean births is to hire a doula. Decades of data confirms that people with doulas have lower rates of Cesarean births. This doesn't mean that doulas are only for people planning to avoid a Cesarean birth—doulas are excellent support for all births—but a doula can help you navigate your choices and advocate for the birth that you'd like.

There are also three types of recommended Cesarean births I want to briefly readdress as areas of possible overuse of Cesarean birth: suspected big babies, obesity, and breech babies. The ACOG states that suspicion of a big baby is not an indication for induction or Cesarean birth (except in very rare cases),[14] but providers continue to routinely counsel patients to consider Cesarean birth for babies on the larger end of normal. The technology used to measure babies in utero only allows estimates within a broad range, and recent studies show many people warned by their provider that their baby was big went on to give birth to a normal-sized baby.[15] If a Cesarean birth is recommended because your baby is suspected to be large, that's a great reason to ask questions, figure out if there are other concerns, get a second opinion, and weigh your options carefully.

Cesarean births are also recommended for and given to large or obese people at much higher rates, and, currently, we don't know why. It's easy to believe our bodies are dangerous and incapable, and many providers assume being larger is a sign of disease or disfunction. I routinely help clients advocate for themselves in a health care system that's deeply fatphobic. Researchers have theories about why large people have more Cesarean births, but we currently don't understand what, if any, connection there is between obesity and labor complications.[16] There may be clinical differences or provider bias, and there definitely seem to be differences in how well technology, like fetal monitoring, functions on large pregnant bodies. Either way, what we *do* know is that large people who have Cesarean births are more likely to have complications afterward and should exercise extra caution in agreeing to a surgical birth. It may be worth questioning the safety of agreeing to a Cesarean birth because of your size alone.

Finally, I want to touch on routine Cesarean birth for breech babies. About 4 percent of babies are in a breech position at thirty-seven weeks, and the best option for delivering those babies vaginally is attempting an external cephalic version (a medical procedure, usually performed in an operating room by a high-risk OB, where they attempt to manually move the baby from a breech position to head down). Knowing the position of your baby before thirty-six weeks is helpful in giving you the option to schedule an external version. Currently less than half of pregnant people with a breech baby attempt a version,[17] many because they're not aware it's an option or not properly counseled on the benefits. While versions don't always work (and success rates vary between practitioners), the average success rate is almost 60 percent.[18] Moreover, the majority of babies successfully turned are then born vaginally. The risks of versions are minimal, but there's a possibility of fetal distress because the umbilical cord is twisted or constricted, in which case you may immediately need a Cesarean birth (one reason versions are often done in operating rooms).

There has also been greater obstetric attention in recent years to the importance of maintaining the skill of delivering breech babies vaginally. For pregnant people who are good candidates for vaginal breech births (only about 30 percent of people with a breech baby fit this description),[19] there is a low risk of complications, and a breech delivery may be a reasonable option. You may be a good candidate for a vaginal breech birth if you:

- Have no contraindications for a vaginal birth
- Have never had a Cesarean birth
- Are at least thirty-six weeks pregnant
- Have a baby estimated to weigh more than 4 pounds and less than about 9.5 pounds
- Have a baby in a frank or complete breech position
- Have a baby with no concerning fetal anomalies
- Are in spontaneous labor

- Are in a facility with skilled staff capable of a breech delivery
- Are in a facility with the ability to perform an emergency Cesarean[20]

If your baby has not moved into a head-down position, you believe you meet these criteria, and you are interested in a vaginal breech birth, searching for a local care provider who is skilled in breech delivery and willing to take you on as a new patient may help you avoid a scheduled Cesarean birth.

THE RISKS OF CESAREAN BIRTH

In many situations, the benefits of a Cesarean birth are profound and lifesaving. Cesarean births, performed for any reason, are considered relatively safe procedures although, absent a significant clinical reason, they pose more risks than a vaginal birth. There are risks of infection, damage to the organs around your uterus (primarily the bladder), heavy bleeding, blood clots in the legs or lungs, and more minor problems like nausea, vomiting, headaches, and constipation. Very rarely, Cesarean birth can be fatal (as can birth more generally, but again, this is a very small risk). There are also some risks to the baby, including injury during surgery and problems associated with being born prematurely (when Cesarean birth happens before thirty-nine weeks or the due date is miscalculated). There are slightly higher long-term risks associated with a Cesarean birth including uterine rupture on the incision scar, future placental problems, and hysterectomy.

As I said, Cesarean births are relatively safe—I don't want to create unwarranted fear—but it's important to be aware of the risks. In the course of my work, I've encountered many people who've incorrectly described Cesarean birth as safer than vaginal birth. This is not true. There are, of course, specific circumstances where a Cesarean birth is substantially safer, but absent a clinical reason, planning for a vaginal birth is safest.

ADVOCATING FOR GENTLE, FAMILY-CENTERED CESAREAN BIRTH

When Cesarean births are necessary or desirable, you can advocate for a birth that's as gentle and positive an experience as possible. A surgical birth can be a beautiful, affirming experience of bringing your child into the world. Grace remembered the birth of her daughter as a magical day, and it's my hope that your birth—however it happens—is remembered as a special experience.

There have been greater efforts recently to make Cesarean birth as gentle and supportive as possible, and a growing number of surgeons are more willing to shift their routine policies and procedures to help patients have more positive experiences. Simple steps—like letting you view the OR in advance so it's more familiar and less frightening, playing music during your Cesarean birth, and letting you wear your own clothing—can help transform the operating room into a more welcoming place.

Shifting how monitoring is done during surgery can also have dramatic effects. If the pulse oximeter, used to monitor your pulse, is on your foot instead of your hand, this allows far more mobility to touch and hold the baby. Similarly, the electrocardiogram (EKG) leads used to monitor your heart can be placed on your back and sides to make space on your chest for skin-to-skin contact with the baby. These are small changes that can make a big difference.

Changing the sterile draping during Cesarean birth can also make a huge difference. It's routine to have a surgical screen during the Cesarean birth, blocking your view of the birth. More patient-friendly options include offering to lower the screen and raising the head of the table so that the birth can be seen, using a clear surgical drape, or using a surgical screen with a flap the baby can be passed through. That said, for some people the idea of seeing their Cesarean birth is wholly unappealing and it's also ok to ask not to have any of these things done.

During the birth, a gentler baby-led approach is possible when there's no distress or urgency. Some surgeons are practicing a slower and more hands-off approach to Cesarean birth. After the head is delivered through the abdominal incision, a pause can allow the baby to begin breathing while still attached to the placenta. Pressure from the uterus can mimic the squeeze babies typically get during a vaginal delivery. The newborn's shoulders can be eased out, pausing again to let uterine contractions (or assistance from the doctor) bring the baby out. This slowed-down birth is a nice approach to surgical delivery in cases where there's no emergency.

There are pediatricians present at Cesarean births, but if your baby is doing well, having your baby immediately skin to skin may be something you'd prefer. Nurses have required newborn tasks such as weighing your baby, administering medications like vitamin K or erythromycin (as required or requested), and taking footprints. Ideally, these can be delayed in favor of you having contact with your baby. Some hospitals have prohibitions against babies being skin to skin in the OR, so ask in advance. If having your baby on your chest isn't possible, hold your baby cheek to cheek to get skin-to-skin contact during the rest

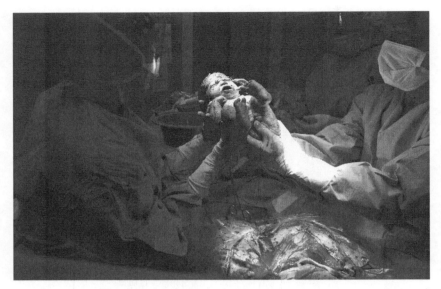

Newborn in a Cesarean birth.

of the surgery and then have the baby placed on your chest immediately in the recovery room.

One difference between vaginal and Cesarean birth that some people are concerned about is the difference in gut bacteria, or "microbiome." Babies are born with sterile intestinal tracts. They develop their gut bacteria, crucial for their immune systems, through exposure to bacteria such as vaginal bacteria, bacteria from skin-to-skin contact, and from chest/breastfeeding.[21] With allergies, asthma, diabetes, and immune system problems increasingly linked to a deficiency of gut bacteria, many worry that a Cesarean birth will limit their baby's microbiome. Some people attempt to "seed" their baby's gut bacteria by swabbing their vaginal fluids prior to birth with a piece of gauze and then wiping this gauze on their baby's face after a Cesarean birth. There are possible concerns about seeding, so speak with your provider about your health and you plans if you're considering this.

Finally, whenever medically possible, keeping your baby with you during surgery and the initial postpartum period in recovery is often something parents desire. Having time to learn to chest/breastfeed or bottle-feed, to cuddle and admire your baby, and to transition together as a family can help create a positive experience. Some hospitals routinely separate healthy babies from their parents, so if nonseparation is important to you, ensure that the place where you're giving birth will respect your preference to stay together.

BIRTHING VIA CESAREAN

The unpredictability of birth was central in Zoe's experience of meeting her son. After multiple miscarriages, she finally had a pregnancy that stuck. She had a doctor she trusted and a hospital she felt confident about. And then, early one warm May morning a few days before her estimated due date, contractions started. She paced the house alone, timing them for a bit before waking her husband, who immediately got to work installing their air conditioners in case she wanted them during labor. I joined them a few hours later. She called the doctors to check in, and the person on call told her to come in anytime she was ready. I reminded her to breathe low and long, and eventually, when Zoe was ready, we headed to the hospital.

The next bit happened quickly: the car ride to the hospital, check-in, monitoring in triage, and a cervical exam that revealed she was 3 cm dilated (not happy news). The doctor suggested Zoe walk around for a few hours before being admitted, but as they were preparing to send her away, the baby's heart rate dropped. She had a deceleration—a big one—and this changed the plans. No more walking: they wanted to keep her and continue monitoring her baby.

Some decelerations are completely normal during labor. Others indicate that the baby is in distress. Zoe's baby had decelerations, large ones, every few hours that would bring everyone running into the room to move her and try to bring the heart rate back up. She couldn't leave the bed or move much because they needed to keep the baby on the monitors. She got an epidural to help her stay still and as a safety precaution in case one of these decelerations prompted an emergency Cesarean. She progressed well—3 cm, 5 cm, 7 cm, and finally 9 cm—but periodically the steady *whoosh-whoosh* of the heart-rate monitor would slow way down.

When the baby's heart rate would go back up, the staff would leave again, and Zoe would wait to see if the *whoosh-whoosh* would hold steady or slow again. She described it as wonderful and horrible—wonderful to be close to meeting their son and horrible to hear the heartbeat go down and worry he might be in trouble. She recalled feeling on edge, waiting for the worst, hoping for the best.

The final deceleration came late that night. This one required a flip onto her hands and knees and medicine to stop her contractions and give the baby time to recover. She was clear: she wanted her baby to be healthy, and she didn't want to hear his heart go down to a slow whisper again. She wanted him out and cared for now. When the doctor came in and gingerly explained to Zoe that she thought it was likely going to be necessary to have a Cesarean birth, Zoe started crying. The doctor assumed she was crying because she didn't want a Cesarean birth. This wasn't at all the case: she was crying from relief. She'd wanted as few interventions in this birth as possible, but faced with the opportunity to have a major surgery and ensure that her distressed baby was born safely, she readily agreed to a Cesarean birth. The doctor took a moment to catch up—moving from apologizing that a Cesarean might be necessary to accepting a high five from Zoe who said, "Let's do this!"

Zoe told me that she understands why some people struggle after an unwanted Cesarean birth, but she could not feel better about her birth. She had a birth team she felt confident in, who treated her with respect and kindness throughout the experience, and she never felt that decisions were being made out of convenience rather than necessity. She told me that Cesareans are not the enemy of a beautiful birth, and she is grateful for her own complicated, beautiful birth.

If your baby is born in a Cesarean birth, it may be an experience you feel wonderful about, like Zoe, or it may take time to come to terms with that experience. Give yourself time to form your own thoughts about your experience and to talk about it when you're ready. It's OK to be upset if your birth did not go as you hoped. Feeling sad or angry doesn't take away from also feeling grateful. You can be both. If you know others who've had Cesarean births, honor and respect their experience of birth.

Stephanie described birthing her son, stating, "If it had happened another way, that might also have been a really great experience but in the end, my son knew what he needed, and I happily gave him that in a cold, sterile OR on the happiest day of my life."

WHAT TO DO WHEN A BABY TURNS BREECH

The standard of care in the US is a Cesarean birth if a baby is breech. Giving birth vaginally is certainly not impossible, but few providers support vaginal breech births (and even those providers prefer babies be head down). Remember that almost all babies will turn head down (vertex) by full term, so if your baby is breech earlier in the pregnancy, this is likely temporary. I recommend clients start really paying attention to position around thirty-two weeks.

- *Confirm it. Sometimes people believe their baby is breech, but they're not. Before you work to move your baby, confirm with your provider that your baby is breech.*

Many people have success encouraging their baby to move into a more optimal position with simple at-home techniques that you and your birth partner can work on together. For example:

- Try shining a flashlight low on your belly to see if the baby is drawn toward the light. You can also play music or have your birth partner talk or sing to your lower belly.
- Try putting cold packs (like frozen peas) on the top of your belly (where the baby's head is) to encourage them to move away from the cold, turning head down.
- Get in a swimming pool and try doing handstands or somersault-like flips underwater to encourage the baby to move.

- Find a safe place to get into a breech tilt position (a Google search will provide hundreds of images to guide you) and do this frequently until the baby flips.
- Try inversions, getting your butt above your head to help encourage the baby to move (again, a Google search will provide lots of examples).
- Trying sleeping on your side with a peanut ball between your legs.

Beyond at-home techniques, speak with your provider about treatment from alternative providers such as an **acupuncturist** or a **chiropractor** to help turn a breech baby. Many people have had success turning their baby using one or both of these techniques.

Also speak with your provider about an **external cephalic version** (or "version") to manually turn the baby into a vertex position.

If your baby **turns vertex** from any of these efforts, stop doing inversions or flips and start doing things to encourage the baby to move lower into your pelvis like sitting cross-legged on the floor, squats, lunges, and walking.

If your baby **remains breech**, then it's time to make plans for a Cesarean birth or a vaginal breech birth, if the option exists locally and you are interested in it.

PLANNING A CESAREAN BIRTH

WHO WILL DELIVER YOUR BABY?

If you are with a doctor who is a solo practitioner, there isn't the same question of who will perform your Cesarean. If you are seeing a midwife or you see care providers in a group practice, then navigating who will be delivering your baby is important.

- If you're seeing midwives, who will they be transferring your care to? When will you meet with them? If they are not a good match, what are your other options?
- If you are seeing a group practice, do you have a preference for one care provider? Are they available to perform your Cesarean? If you end up needing to give birth before your scheduled Cesarean, will this care provider still be able to support you?

WHO WILL SUPPORT YOU DURING YOUR BIRTH?

Between your preferences and hospital policy, determine who can be with you before, during, and after your birth to support you physically and emotionally, help you care for the baby, and chest/breastfeed or bottle-feed.

- How many support people are you allowed to have with you before your Cesarean?
- How many support people can you have in the operating room with you?
- How many support people can you have with you in recovery and in your postpartum room during the days after your birth? Can they stay overnight?
- Who would you like with you at each of these stages (and are there people you'd like to make sure are not there)?
- If you do not have any support people you'd like to have with you, is there a nurse or a medical student or other staff member of the hospital who can support you as needed?

WHO ELSE WILL BE THERE?

Cesarean births are major surgery, and as such, there will be a large team of doctors, nurses, and hospital staff. Knowing who will be with you during your birth and what to expect in the operating room can be reassuring.

- Who will be assisting your doctor (an additional doctor, a resident, medical students)?
- Who else will be with you (anesthesiologists, pediatricians, nurses, other staff)?
- How will you interact with the other people in the room, if at all, during your birth?

PREFERENCES FOR THE BIRTH

While there are some things about any birth that you can't control, you can have preferences for your birth even if your birth is in an operating room.

- Would you like your doctor to explain to you what is happening, or would you prefer the conversation to be about something other than the Cesarean?

- Do you want music playing in the operating room or other forms of distraction?
- Would you prefer a clear drape or to have the drape lowered so you can see the birth?
- How soon after the birth can you hold the baby? Can you have your baby skin to skin if you'd like?
- If you can't hold the baby (or prefer not to), can your partner or support person hold the baby in the operating room?
- Can nonurgent newborn procedures be delayed until after you hold your baby?
- Can they put the EKG monitors on your back and pulse ox on your toe to make holding the baby on your chest easier?
- Are there other preferences you have for your Cesarean birth?

CONCLUSION
Birthing Unapologetically

As I began writing this book, I pitched the idea to other birth professionals: doulas, doctors, midwives, nurses, therapists. The responses were generous and appreciated, but the greatest resistance came from older midwives. One midwife said she was "squirming" reading that I didn't use the words "natural birth," because "there is truly a difference between natural birth and one hooked up to machines." Another midwife told me someone who elected a Cesarean birth and considered it a positive experience "had poor informed choice and no one put her fear of labor pain in perspective with the reality of surgery and post-operative pain."

While I respect both of these midwives tremendously, I disagree. It's true that birth is different with or without monitors and medications. It is also true that Cesareans are major surgery. That said, I don't agree that one way is better or worse. You might have a really positive Cesarean birth that you choose, and you shouldn't have to defend that decision against those who'd say this isn't a choice you can thoughtfully make. These midwives wanted to be supportive of me but didn't feel comfortable with my assertion that a positive birth wasn't a particular type of birth experience or outcome.

I believe part of this conflict is generational. They came into birth work closer to a time when the medical model of birth still routinely included things like twilight sleep to reduce pain while causing amnesia, Pitocin to prompt contractions, episiotomies and forceps for delivery in an operating room with no support people, and almost no choices or attention to consent. This medicalization of birth gave rise to a natural childbirth movement that offered alternatives for people like my mother who wanted to give birth without pain medication or other drugs, with the support of her partner, and outside of an operating room.

These midwives dedicated their lives to changing birth so that people like me and you could give birth in more compassionate, more respectful, more present, and more informed ways. I'm thankful for this. And yet, their response to my pitch is precisely why I wrote this book.

You've likely heard the expression "Don't throw the baby out with the bathwater," a warning to not get rid of something valuable while trying to eliminate something undesired. I'm reminded of this. In an effort to change birth so that pregnant people had more control, more choices, more support, and real opportunities to give consent or refuse treatment, there might have been some overcorrecting. The goal shouldn't be to create another, oppositional model of birth to dictate what everyone should want or do. It's no more empowering for me or a midwife or a doctor or someone else to tell you what choices to make or what you should want. The goal is for pregnant people to make informed, autonomous choices in childbirth.

Making an informed choice about your birth doesn't mean someone gives you the information they want you to have so you'll make the choice they want you to make. It means having all the information, without agenda or opinion. It means being empowered to make your own choices. This is what I have aimed to do here.

In over a decade of doing this work, I have seen such a huge variety of positive births planned to the vision of very different people who wanted very different things from their birth experiences. Your way might be a quiet hospital room with just you and your partner moving through contractions together in what feels like a very intimate and private moment in your lives. Your way might be a homebirth with a dozen friends and family members gathered around making food and music and giving you love while you labor. Your way might be your best friend, who donated his sperm to help you become a mother, crying on FaceTime from across the country as he heads to the airport to come take care of you in your first weeks postpartum. Your way might be your dog curled up on your lap, not sure what to make of the sounds you're making, but offering you warmth and love all the same. Your way might be your sisters, who live nearby, showing up with soup and toilet paper and hugs, ready to be your birth partners as you head into single parenthood. Your way might be an induction, a Cesarean, a midwife, a water birth, an operating room, a high-risk doctor, nitrous oxide, a back rub. This is *your* birth.

I do this work because I believe birth matters. The physical and emotional experience of giving birth is both memorable and significant in our lives. Having an experience of coming into parenthood that you feel good about, whatever that looks like, matters. It's my hope that you'll take the information here and use it to unapologetically plan a birth experience that matches your desires. Whatever you want, wherever you are, however it happens: this is your birth. I hope it's a positive experience.

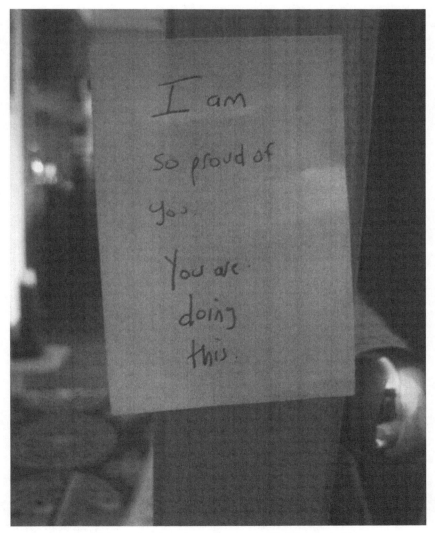

Sticky note written by a partner at a birth I attended.

UNDERSTANDING COMMON NEWBORN PROCEDURES

VITAMIN K

Newborns have low levels of vitamin K, needed for clotting blood. Giving an injection of vitamin K after birth prevents a rare but potentially fatal bleeding disorder called vitamin K deficiency bleeding (VKDB). Vitamin K shots have routinely been given in the US to newborns since 1961 but are only mandatory in a few states.

- Is vitamin K mandatory at the birth location you have chosen?
- If it is not mandatory, can you request that your baby be given a vitamin K shot?

ERYTHROMYCIN OINTMENT

Antibacterial ointment is placed in newborns' eyes as prophylaxis against ophthalmia neonatorum, a type of eye infection contracted during birth, primarily from undiagnosed chlamydia or gonorrhea (sexually transmitted infections). Reported adverse effects include eye irritation and blurred vision and the small possibility that it contributes to antibiotic-resistant bacteria. This treatment is mandatory in most states.

- Is erythromycin ointment mandatory at the birth location you have chosen?

- Were you tested for chlamydia/gonorrhea during the pregnancy? What were the results?
- If it's not mandatory, can you request treatment with erythromycin?

HEPATITIS B VACCINE

The hepatitis B vaccine is given to prevent a life-threatening liver infection that can be transmitted to children if they're bitten by an infected person, touch the open wounds of an infected person, share a toothbrush with an infected person, or eat food chewed by an infected person. It can also be transmitted during birth and later in life, during sex or IV drug use. If you have hepatitis B, the recommendation is that your baby be treated with an additional medication in the first twelve hours of life. If you don't have hepatitis B, the recommendation is to have the first dose of the vaccine administered during the first day of life (and additional doses later in infancy) to protect against future infection. Vaccines are not currently mandatory.

- Is the hepatitis B vaccine administered at the birth location you have chosen?
- Does your pediatrician provide the hepatitis B vaccine in their office as an alternative to receiving the vaccine at the birth location?

NEWBORN SCREENING

A small sample of blood is collected from a newborn's heel within a few days of birth and is used to screen for rare genetic, endocrine, and metabolic disorders. This test allows for early detection and treatment. Newborn screenings vary greatly between states. A hearing test and a test for critical congenital heart defects can also be administered. Some tests may not be available at your birth location and will require follow-up elsewhere.

- What tests are administered at your birth location?
- If not all tests are available, where can you follow up to get these tests for your baby?

• Who will follow up with you about the results of the newborn screening?

BLOOD SUGAR TESTING

Small babies, large babies, babies born to someone with gestational diabetes, and babies in the NICU are routinely tested for low blood sugar in the hours and days after birth. Different birth locations and providers have different policies for what counts as small and large, as well as how often and for how long after the birth blood sugar tests are required. These tests involve a needle prick to the newborn's heel, pushing a drop of blood out, and using a blood glucose reader to get a plasma glucose level for your baby.

• What are the policies for blood sugar readings at your birth location?
• Can you hold your baby while the blood sugar tests are administered?
• If your baby has low blood sugar, how will they help bring the blood sugar levels up (skin to skin, chest/breastfeeding, glucose gel, supplementing with pumped milk or formula, etc.)?

CIRCUMCISION

The foreskin covers the head (glans) of the penis. A circumcision is the surgical removal of this skin, usually performed in the first days of life by an OB, a pediatrician, or a religious practitioner such as a mohel. When performed in the hospital, circumcisions are typically done apart from the parents but a pediatrician or mohel may perform the circumcision with you present. The procedure usually takes about ten minutes followed by several days of keeping the penis covered with ointment and gauze to heal. Circumcisions have long been performed for cultural and religious reasons in many areas of the word, but the US is one of the only countries where nonreligious circumcisions are routinely performed. In the US, circumcision rates vary between regions, races, religion, and insurance coverage. Reported benefits to circumcision include fewer UTIs, lower rates of penile cancer, and a reduction in HIV and HPV acquisition. Reported risks include procedure-related complications (surgical error, infection, bleeding, adhesions, etc.), sexual dissatisfaction or pain, and potential breast-feeding troubles. While circumcisions were once routinely recommended, most health organizations in the US say that the medical benefits alone do not justify routine circumcisions and parents should weigh the risks and benefits with their own beliefs and preferences when making a decision.

- Do you have questions about choosing to have or not have a circumcision performed?
- Who will perform it? How many circumcisions have they performed? How do you make arrangements for it? Will you be present with your baby when it happens?
- Is there an additional cost associated, or will insurance cover the procedure?
- Is there any anesthetic (pain-relieving medication) given to your baby before or after the circumcision? If so, what types?
- What special care will your baby require while healing? Who will teach you the wound care techniques you need to know?
- If you do not have a circumcision performed, how can you minimize risks with good hygiene? Can your pediatrician help you teach your child to wash beneath their foreskin regularly after it is fully retractable?

NAVIGATING THE NICU

The NICU can be an overwhelming place. No one likes to see their baby attached to machines and monitors, and whatever the circumstances that brought you there, it's never anyone's first choice. You might know in advance that your baby will likely spend time in the NICU, or it might be a surprise. If you know in advance, it can be great to ask questions and prepare yourself as much as possible. Either way, here are some tips to help navigate your time in the NICU and make that as positive an experience as possible.

WRITE IT DOWN

As soon as possible, start taking notes. If there is someone you can ask to help with this, like a doula or family member, delegate the job. Ask for names; write down tests, any diagnosis made, and your concerns. Start making lists of questions so you can get answers from the right people when they're available. Find out how you can speak to your baby's team and get updates even if you're not there. Find out the feeding schedule for your baby or when other important things are scheduled to happen. This can also act as a journal if you are someone who could benefit from journaling as an outlet for all the feelings you might be having.

DO NOT BE AFRAID TO ASK QUESTIONS

No one wants to put their baby at risk, so it's easy to feel intimidated by the suggestions given to you in a NICU, but you should feel free to question everything, get a second opinion if desired, talk through the treatment plan, and discuss the recommendations as much as you need. You are your baby's advocate, and asking questions can help you make the best decisions about their care.

LEARN THE TITLES

Hospital hierarchies are rarely familiar unless you work in a hospital (or watch a lot of hospital-based TV dramas). There will be a team of neonatologists (doctors trained to work in the NICU specifically), and they'll often have a team of fellows, residents, and medical students who work with them. If you're not clear on what's being recommended or you don't agree with the recommendation, sometimes speaking to the neonatologist can be clarifying or allow you to negotiate a new plan. There will also be nurses and nurse practitioners you'll likely interact with the most. They are most centrally involved in caring for your baby and can often be an excellent advocate for you and your baby. You might also meet a variety of therapists (physical, respiratory) and social workers.

GET INVOLVED

It's easy to be intimidated by tubes and wires attached to your baby, but it is so valuable for you and your baby to spend as much time as you can skin to skin. Having your baby on your chest (or someone else's chest) will help your baby get healthy and stay healthy, getting you all home faster. Also, talk to the nurses about helping with diaper changes, bathing, feeding, and caring for your baby. Nurses are often wonderful at teaching you all sorts of parenting skills that will be super helpful for when you leave.

IF YOU ARE PLANNING TO CHEST/BREASTFEED

Get a hospital-grade double electric pump right away. Hospitals often have one you can use while you're there, and they also often rent them if you'd like to have one at home. Find out where you can store your milk for your baby and what you need to do to label it. Ask to meet with the lactation consultant, if there is one, or see one privately. Advocate for your baby getting as much milk as soon as possible (and be prepared to have to ask for this repeatedly since it's not uncommon for there to be a lot of pressure to give formula in the NICU). Your hospital might have access to donor human milk if you don't have milk yet or your supply is not enough. Ask the nurses what's available.

REMEMBER IT TAKES TIME

Hospitals can be very slow and frustrating places. It's common for things to happen more slowly than expected and for totally unrealistic time frames to be suggested. Someone might say they'll be back in fifteen minutes and never return. A procedure might be scheduled for 8:00 a.m. but happen in the afternoon. Be prepared for this. Also, expect there to be setbacks and some disappointment on the road to getting out of the NICU. This can be an emotional roller coaster, and being prepared for it can lessen the impact.

TAKE CARE OF YOURSELF

Depending on the hospital you are in, the accommodations for parents with a baby in the NICU might be very nice or incredibly minimal. If you know you'll need to spend time in the NICU in advance, it's great to research your options. No matter what the conditions, make sure you keep hydrated, eat meals, and find the coziest place to hang out with your baby. You have the right to be with your baby 24/7, but you should make sure you make time to sleep every day. You might also benefit from the support of other parents who have babies in the NICU currently or who've lived through the experience already. Finding online or in-person support groups can be helpful.

CHEST/BREASTFEEDING BASICS AND SIGNS YOU MIGHT NEED HELP

If your plan is to nurse, it's helpful to know what to expect and when to get help. Many people have heard negative stories about chest/breastfeeding, and this can be intimidating. The majority of people have a lot of success, and getting help early can really increase your odds of success.

WHAT TO EXPECT

Frequency

Babies nurse a lot and need food around the clock. Most recommendations say to feed every two to three hours, but it's not uncommon for a baby to want to nurse more than that. They can digest a stomach full of milk quickly and might cluster a number of feeds close together. They will also occasionally sleep a bit longer than this, especially as they get older.

Duration

My clients are often overwhelmed by conflicting advice on how long they should expect to be feeding. Duration alone is usually not a great marker of how well feeding is going. Some babies nurse vigorously and transfer all the milk they need quickly. Other babies might chest/breastfeed for hours but hardly transfer any milk at all. Given this, while it can be useful to have a sense of how long your baby is nursing for on average, I don't recommend you focus too much on duration if everything else looks good.

Switching Sides

Many people worry they'll need to keep close track of which side their baby is nursing from. While it might feel better for you if you nurse in approximately even amounts, stressing about starting on the left or the right at each feed is unnecessary.

Weight

It's normal, and expected, for your baby to lose some weight in the beginning (up to 10 percent of their birth weight is normal). After an initial weight loss in the first days, your baby should begin to gain weight, getting back up to their birth weight within a couple weeks.

Tracking

There are a number of apps and paper forms you can use to track the frequency and duration of feeds and when your baby has a wet or soiled diaper. This information can be useful in the first week, especially in communicating with a lactation consultant or pediatrician. Once chest/breastfeeding is going well and your baby is gaining weight, you can stop tracking.

SIGNS OF SUCCESS

Things are going well if your baby is nursing frequently, pooping and peeing often (usually this means at least five to six wet diapers a day), gaining weight (your pediatrician will confirm this), and you are feeling increasingly confident and positive about chest/breastfeeding.

YOU MIGHT NEED HELP

If you are in a lot of pain while feeding, if your baby is not pooping or peeing often, if your baby is losing weight or not gaining weight at the expected rate, or if you feel like you are not gaining confidence and could use help with positioning, technique, or information, it is time to reach out to a local lactation consultant or La Leche League for more support.

TAKING CARE OF YOURSELF

Remember that nursing is something you will do repeatedly throughout the day, often for months (maybe years), so finding strategies to be comfortable when you feed your baby and making sure you stay hydrated and well fed can be key to having a positive nursing experience.

Having a comfortable chair, lots of pillows to support your baby and your arms, a nearby table with water and snacks, and easy access to things like your phone, ebook reader, or remote can make it even nicer to nurse (and potentially have a baby sleep on your chest after feeding).

PREPARING FOR POSTPARTUM

The postpartum experience is widely varied, but for many people, it's much harder than they imagined it would be. You might be more uncomfortable, more hormonal, more exhausted, more overwhelmed, and more thirsty and hungry than you've ever been before! I cried in the shower because the water was warm. We had dinner at 11:00 p.m. because we couldn't get it together to eat sooner. I seemed to always have milk or spit-up or baby pee on my clothes. And doing all of that while wearing a giant menstrual pad around the clock was terrible. I could write a book on postpartum and parenting, but for now, here are a few tips to help you prepare.

THINGS TO HAVE ON HAND

No matter how you give birth, you'll want to have pads for postpartum bleeding (expect to bleed for several weeks, most heavily in the beginning and tapering off). There are lots of online recommendations for soaking and freezing pads to wear afterward, but be careful about putting frozen pads on your tender tissue as you might do more harm than good. You might also want to have over-the-counter pain medications like Motrin and Tylenol on hand and a stool softener, like Colace. Speak with your provider about these. Most hospitals and birth centers (and your homebirth kit) will include a peri bottle, used to spray water on your healing genitals. The peri bottle can be used to dilute your urine when you pee if you find it stings when you urinate, and it can be used to clean away urine and blood. You'll also see a lot of recommendations for sitz baths, herbs, sprays, and you might find some of these things helpful, but I wouldn't put them on an essentials list per se.

It's great to have tons of nutrient-dense snacks and lots of options for keeping yourself well fed. Maybe friends or family are bringing you snacks and meals, or you've stocked your pantry and freezer? Or, maybe you'll be getting more takeout and delivery? Additionally, most people enjoy having a water bottle or sealed cup nearby them to stay hydrated. Between blood loss, making milk (if you are), and night sweats, most people need to drink a lot.

TASKS YOU MIGHT NEED HELP WITH

It'll likely be difficult for you to make meals, do laundry, and help with housecleaning, grocery shopping, or other errands. If these aren't tasks you routinely did before giving birth, then this might not be a big adjustment. If these are tasks you did, it'll be helpful to plan for someone else to do these things for several weeks. If you're someone who's used to getting a lot done every day, it might be hard to recognize how difficult it can be to accomplish as many things as you used to. You will be healing and taking care of a newborn, which is far more work than a full-time job for most people. You might have friends, family, a doula, a newborn care specialist (night nanny), a cleaning service, or others helping you. You might also look into local grocery and meal delivery or laundry services.

For many of us, it's hard to ask for help even if we're totally overwhelmed and badly need help. For some people, they do better hiring people to help than asking friends or family. For others, counting on friends and family is more ideal, and it's just a matter of getting over a reluctance to ask for help. This could mean making a list of things you need done and sharing it with friends and family, or it could mean making plans in advance to have people do specific tasks for you.

You might need help holding your baby sometimes, especially while you eat, sleep, or take a shower. That said, for most people, help holding a baby isn't the most critical help. Maybe people have imagined having a parent or sibling around postpartum will mean they're well cared for, only to discover the person wasn't very helpful. Make sure your imagined helpers are really prepared to be helpers and are planning to do things like dishes and errands (and not just hold the baby). Also, consider warning people in advance that you'd like the option to politely kick people out if you are feeling overwhelmed or preferring privacy.

CARING FOR YOURSELF

You should expect to not leave your house for a couple of weeks (except doctor's appointments) in order to heal. No matter how you gave birth, you're healing from the wound where your placenta was and from the pregnancy itself. On top of this, you might be healing from a vaginal laceration or a Cesarean incision, blood loss, hemorrhoids, or injury to your pelvis. Make sure you know what exactly happened to your body, how best to heal and care for yourself, and how to be as comfortable as possible. Seeing a pelvic floor physical therapist postpartum can also be very helpful.

When I gave birth I was both profoundly exhausted and also filled with hormones that had me (irrationally) wanting to be out doing things. I highly recommend you do everything possible to fight this urge and stay home for at least a couple of weeks. Prioritize sleeping instead. You'll hear everyone tell you to sleep when the baby sleeps, and this is true, but also just sleep anytime you can. A face mask, earplugs, dark curtains, or a fan might help you rest during odd hours.

I highly recommend finding a supportive community for yourself. This could be a new parent group (online or in person), a chest/breastfeeding circle, or a group of friends you already had. Being a new parent can be lonely, scary, and isolating. Having people who understand what you are going through and are supportive can be a game changer. Consider asking someone who loves you unconditionally to check in every day. Be honest with them about where you are.

A note on sex: you don't get "cleared for sex" by a doctor or midwife after you give birth, even if your provider has incorrectly suggested this is something they'll do. In the immediate weeks after birth, it's best to avoid vaginal penetrative sex while you're healing (both healing from stitches but also your cervix and uterus). After you're healed, you can have (or not have) sex anytime you'd like. No one needs to clear you for this except *you*, and no one gets to determine when that is—not your provider or your partner or anyone else. Be gentle with yourself, consider using lots of lube, try things that don't require penetration to start, and stop anytime if you find you aren't enjoying it.

A note about your body: Your body will be different immediately postpartum and it may be different forever (and this could be in ways you love or ways you're learning to accept). You might be heavier, have more skin on your belly, have stretch marks or scars. The cultural narrative about "getting your body back" or "bouncing back" is so destructive and unreasonable. You made a human being and birthed them from your body. It is OK if that changed you. You do not need to get your body back; it has always been with you and it will remain with you, in whatever shape that is currently.

If you feel like you're getting too overwhelmed, too exhausted, or you're feeling emotionally not OK, please find help. This could be a local therapist or doctor, a postpartum doula, a support group, or an online forum for postpartum people or specifically for postpartum depression or other postpartum mood disorders, among other resources. It can be really hard to tell people that you're not OK, but there is so much more awareness and support for new parents today. I hope you'll utilize these resources so you can start feeling better. Also, it's OK to feel like maybe you made a huge mistake. That does not make you a bad parent, but it might be a good sign that you need a nap and some more support.

NOTES

INTRODUCTION

1. Childbirth Connection, "Quick Facts about Labor Induction," National Partnership for Women and Families Fact Sheet, August 2016; William Grobman, "Induction of Labor with Oxytocin," in *UpToDate*, ed. Ted W. Post (Waltham, MA: UpToDate, 2018); Michelle J. K. Osterman and Joyce A. Martin, "Recent Declines in Induction of Labor by Gestational Age," *NCHS Data Brief*, no. 155 (June 2014).

2. Meaghan A. Leddy, Michael L. Power, and Jay Schulkin, "The Impact of Maternal Obesity on Maternal and Fetal Health," *Obstetrics & Gynecology* 1, no. 4 (2008): 170–78; Megan Davidson and Sarah Lewin, "Eating for Two: The Fear and Threat of Fatness in Pregnancy," in *Heavy Burdens: Stories of Motherhood and Fatness*, ed. Judy Verseghy and Sam Abel (Bradford, ON: Demeter, 2018); Megan Davidson and Sarah Lewin, "Dangerous Bodies: Imagining, Monitoring, and Managing Fatness during Pregnancy," in *Bearing the Weight of the World: Exploring Maternal Embodiment*, ed. Alys Einion and Jen Rinaldi (Bradford, ON: Demeter, 2018).

3. Nina Martin and Renee Montagne, "Lost Mothers: Nothing Protects Black Women from Dying in Pregnancy and Childbirth. Not Education. Not Income, Not Even Being an Expert on Racial Disparities in Health," *Propublica*, December 7, 2017, https://www.propublica.org/article/nothing-protects-black-women-from-dying-in-pregnancy-and-childbirth; Laura Villarosa, "Why American's Black Mothers and Babies Are in a Life-or-Death Crisis: The Answer to the Disparity in Death Rates Has Everything to Do with the Lived Experience of Being a Black Woman in America," *New York Times Magazine*, April 11, 2018, https://www.nytimes.com/2018/04/11/magazine/black-mothers-babies-death-maternal-mortality.html.

4. Luis Ferre-Sadurni, "New York to Expand Use of Doulas to Reduce Childbirth Deaths," *New York Times*, April 22, 2018, https://www.nytimes.com/2018/04/22/nyregion/childbirth-death-doula-medicaid.html.

CHAPTER 2

1. "Birth and Natality," National Center for Health Statistics, last updated March 31, 2017, https://www.cdc.gov/nchs/fastats/births.htm; Marian MacDorman, T. J. Mathews, and Eugene Declercq, "Trends in Out-of-Hospital Births in the United States, 1990–2012," *NCHS Data Brief*, no. 144 (March 2014): 1.

2. "Maternity Length of Stay Rules," National Conference of State Legislatures, April 23, 2018, http://www.ncsl.org/research/health/final-maternity-length-of-stay-rules-published.aspx.

3. Tara Haelle, "Your Biggest C-Section Risk May Be Your Hospital: Consumer Reports Finds That Your Odds of Having a C-Section Can Be over Nine Times Higher If You Pick the Wrong Hospital," *Consumer Reports*, May 10, 2018, https://www.consumerreports.org/c-section/biggest-c-section-risk-may-be-your-hospital/.

CHAPTER 3

1. Kitty Ernst and Kate Bauer, "Birth Centers in the United States," American Association of Birth Centers, 2017, 10, https://cdn.ymaws.com/www.birthcenters.org/resource/collection/028792A7-808D-4BC7-9A0F-FB038B434B91/Birth_Center_in_the_United_States.pdf.

2. Marian MacDorman and Eugene Declercq, "Trends and Characteristics of United States Out-of-Hospital Births 2004–2014: New Information on Risk Status and Access of Care," *Birth: Issues in Perinatal Care* 43, no. 2 (June 2016): 116–24; Marian F. Mac-Dorman, T. J. Mathews, and Eugene Declercq, "Trends in Out-of-Hospital Births in the United States, 1990–2012," *NCHS Data Brief*, no. 144 (March 2014), https://www.cdc.gov/nchs/data/databriefs/db144.htm#x2013;2012</a>%20.

3. Ernst and Bauer, "Birth Centers," 10; Phil Galewitz, "Not a Hospital, Not a Home Birth: The Rise of the Birth Center," CNN, October 12, 2015, https://www.cnn.com/2015/10/12/health/us-birth-centers-increase/index.html.

4. Rebecca Dekker, "Evidence Confirms Birth Centers Provide Top-Notch Care," American Association of Birth Centers, January 31, 2013, https://www.birthcenters.org/page/NBCSII?#cost-savings.

5. Eugene R. Declercq, Carol Sakala, Maureen P. Corry, Sandra Applebaum, and Ariel Herrlich, "Major Survey Findings of Listening to Mothers (SM) III: Pregnancy and Birth: Report of the Third National U.S. Survey of Women's Childbearing Experiences," *Journal of Perinatal Education* 23, no. 1 (2014): 9–16; Rebecca Dekker, "The Evidence On: Birth Positions," Evidence Based Birth, February 2, 2018, https://evidencebasedbirth.com/evidence-birthing-positions/.

6. S. Bernitz, R. Rolland, E. Blix, M. Jacobsen, K. Sjøborg, and P. Øian, "Is the Operative Delivery Rate in Low-Risk Women Dependent on the Level of Birth Care? A Randomised Controlled Trial," *BJOG* 118, no. 11 (June 12, 2011): 1357; J. T.

Fullerton and R. J. Severino, "In-Hospital Care for Low-Risk Childbirth: Comparison with Results from the National Birth Center Study," *Nurse Midwifery* 37, no. 5 (1992): 331; Susan Stapleton, "Birth Centers," in *UpToDate*, ed. Ted W. Post (Waltham, MA: UpToDate, 2018).

7. Judith P. Rooks, Norman L. Weatherby, Eunice K. Ernst, Susan Stapleton, David Rosen, and Allan Rosenfield, "Outcomes of Care in Birth Centers: The National Birth Center Study," *New England Journal of Medicine* 321, no. 26 (1989): 1804; Judith P. Rooks, Norman L. Weatherby, and Eunice K. Ernst, "The National Birth Center Study: Part III—Intrapartum and Immediate Postpartum and Neonatal Complications and Transfers, Postpartum and Neonatal Care, Outcomes, and Client Satisfaction," *Journal of Nurse Midwifery* 37, no. 6 (1992): 361; Susan Stapleton, C. Osborne, and J. Illuzzi, "Outcomes of Care in Birth Centers: Demonstration of a Durable Model," *Journal of Midwifery & Women's Health* 58, no. 1 (January 30, 2013): 3–14; Stapleton, "Birth Centers."

CHAPTER 4

1. American College of Obstetricians and Gynecologists (ACOG), "Planned Home Birth," *Committee Opinion*, no. 697 (April 2017, reaffirmed 2018), https://www. acog.org/Clinical-Guidance-and-Publications/Committee-Opinions/Committee-on-Obstetric-Practice/Planned-Home-Birth; Debora Boucher, Catherine Bennett, Barbara McFarlin, and Rixa Freeze, "Staying Home to Give Birth: Why Women in the United States Choose Home Birth," *Journal of Midwifery & Women's Health* 54, no. 2 (2009): 119; Marian F. MacDorman, T. J. Mathews, and Eugene Declercq, "Trends in Out-of-Hospital Births in the United States, 1990–2012," *NCHS Data Brief*, no. 144 (March 2014), https://www.cdc.gov/nchs/products/databriefs/db144.htm.

2. ACOG, "Planned Home Birth."

3. ACOG, "Planned Home Birth."

4. Eugene Declercq, Marian F. MacDorman, Fay Menacker, and Naomi Stotland, "Characteristics of Planned and Unplanned Home Births in 19 States," *Obstetrics & Gynecology* 116, no. 1 (July 2010): 95.

PART II

1. Christine Morton and Elayne Clift, *Birth Ambassadors: Doulas and the Re-Emergence of Women-Supported Birth in America* (Amarillo, TX: Praeclarus, 2014); Choices in Childbirth, *Doula Care in NYC: Advancing the Goals of the Affordable Care Act* (New York: Choices in Childbirth, 2014).

CHAPTER 5

1. Joyce A. Martin, Brady E. Hamilton, Michelle J. K. Osterman, Anne K. Driscoll, and Patrick Drake, "Births: Final Data for 2016," *National Vital Statistics Reports* 67, no. 1 (January 31, 2018), https://www.cdc.gov/nchs/data/nvsr/nvsr67/nvsr67_01.pdf.

2. Coco A. Cohen, "Declining Trends in the Provision of Prenatal Care Visits by Family Physicians," *Annuals of Family Medicine* 7 (2009): 128–33; Janelle Guirguis-Blake, Ed Fryer, Mark Deutchman, Larry Green, Susan Dovey, and Robert Phillips, "Family Physicians' Declining Contribution to Prenatal Care in the United States," *American Family Physician*, no. 66 (2002): 2192; Sebastian T. C. Tong, Laura A. Makaroff, Imam M. Xierali, Parwen Parhat, James C. Puffer, Warren P. Newton, and Andrew W. Bazemore, "Proportion of Family Physicians Providing Maternity Care Continues to Decline," *Journal of the American Board of Family Medicine* 25, no. 3 (May–June 2012): 270–71.

CHAPTER 6

1. Judith R. Rooks, "The History of Midwifery: Revised and Updated," Our Bodies Our Selves, May 22, 2014, https://www.ourbodiesourselves.org/book-excerpts/health-article/history-of-midwifery/.

2. Midwifery Task Force, "Midwives Model of Care," National Association of Certified Professional Midwives, accessed June 27, 2017, http://nacpm.org/about-cpms/midwifery-model-of-care/.

3. Midwives Alliance of North America (MANA), "The Midwives Model of Care," accessed November 23, 2018, https://mana.org/about-midwives/midwifery-model.

4. American College of Nurse-Midwives (ACNM), "Essential Facts about Midwives: Midwives & Birth in the United States," accessed July 29, 2017, http://www.midwife.org/Essential-Facts-about-Midwives; National Association of Certified Professional Midwives (NACPM), "Who Are CPMs," accessed July 29, 2017, http://nacpm.org/about-cpms/who-are-cpms/.

5. Phyllis L. Brodsky, "Where Have All the Midwives Gone?," *Journal of Perinatal Education* 17, no. 4 (Fall 2008): 48–51, https://www.ncbi.nlm.nih.gov/pmc/articles/PMC2582410/.

6. ACNM, "Essential Facts about Midwives."

7. NACPM, "Who Are CPMs."

8. North American Registry of Midwives, "Current Status," accessed November 24, 2018, http://narm.org/certification/current-status/.

9. Jane Sandall, Hora Soltani, Simon Gates, Andrew Shennan, and Declan Devane, "Midwife-Led Continuity Models of Care Compared with Other Models of Care for Women during Pregnancy, Birth and Early Parenting," *Cochrane Database of Systematic Reviews*, April 28, 2016, http://www.cochrane.org/CD004667/PREG_midwife-

led-continuity-models-care-compared-other-models-care-women-during-pregnancy-birth-and-early.

10. American College of Obstetricians and Gynecologists (ACOG), "Planned Home Birth," *Committee Opinion*, no. 697 (April 2017, reaffirmed 2018), https://www.acog.org/Clinical-Guidance-and-Publications/Committee-Opinions/Committee-on-Obstetric-Practice/Planned-Home-Birth.

11. American College of Obstetricians and Gynecologists (ACOG), "ACOG Endorses the International Confederation of Midwives Standards for Midwifery Education, Training, Licensure and Regulation," American College of Obstetricians and Gynecologists, April 20, 2015, https://www.acog.org/About-ACOG/News-Room/Statements/2015/ACOG-Endorses-the-International-Confederation-of-Midwives-Standards-for-Midwifery-Education.

CHAPTER 7

1. Dana Raphael, *The Tender Gift: Breastfeeding* (Englewood Cliffs, NJ: Prentice Hall, 1973).

2. Sharon Muza, "Remembering Dr. John Kennell and His Great Contributions to Mothers and Babies Worldwide," *Science & Sensibility*, updated February 2, 2017, accessed September 4, 2018, https://www.scienceandsensibility.org/blog/remembering-dr.-john-kennell-and-his-great-contributions-to-mothers-and-babies-worldwide.

3. Choices in Childbirth, *Doula Care in NYC: Advancing the Goals of the Affordable Care Act* (New York: Choices in Childbirth, 2014); A. Gilliland, "Beyond Holding Hands: The Modern Role of the Professional Doula," *Journal of Obstetrics, Gynecologic, & Neonatal Nursing* 31, no. 6 (November–December 2002): 762–69; Kenneth Gruber, Susan Cupito, and Christina Dobson, "Impact of Doulas on Healthy Birth Outcomes," *Journal of Perinatal Education* 21, no. 1 (Winter 2013): 49–58; Rachel Gurevich, *The Doula Advantage: Your Complete Guide to Having an Empowered and Positive Birth with the Help of a Professional Childbirth Assistant* (New York: Prima, 2003); Meghan A. Bohren, G. Justus Hofmeyr, Carol Sakala, Rieko K. Fukuzawa, and Anna Cuthbert, "Continuous Support for Women during Childbirth," *Cochrane Database of Systematic Reviews*, issue 7, no. CD003766 (2017), https://doi.org/10.1002/14651858.CD003766.pub6; Marshall Klaus, John Kennell, and Phyllis H. Klaus, *The Doula Book*, 3rd ed. (Cambridge, MA: Perseus, 2012); Marshall Klaus, John Kennell, and Phyllis H. Klaus, *Mothering the Mother* (Boston: Addison-Wesley, 1993).

4. Megan Davidson, "Experts in Birth: How Doulas Improve Outcomes for Birthing Women and Their Babies," in *Doulas and Intimate Labour: Boundaries, Bodies and Birth*, ed. Angela N. Castaneda and Julie Johnson Searcy (Bradford, ON: Demeter, 2015), 15–31.

5. American College of Obstetricians and Gynecologists (ACOG) and the Society for Maternal-Fetal Medicine (SMFM), "Safe Prevention of the Primary Cesarean Delivery," *Obstetric Care Consensus*, no. 1 (March 2014, reaffirmed 2016): 13.

6. Christine Morton and Elayne Clift, *Birth Ambassadors: Doulas and the Re-emergence of Women-Supported Birth in America* (Amarillo, TX: Praeclarus, 2014); Choices in Childbirth, *Doula Care in NYC: Advancing the Goals of the Affordable Care Act* (New York: Choices in Childbirth, 2014).

CHAPTER 8

1. American College of Obstetricians and Gynecologists (ACOG) and the Society for Maternal-Fetal Medicine (SMFM), "Safe Prevention of the Primary Cesarean Delivery," *Obstetric Care Consensus*, no. 1 (March 2014, reaffirmed 2016): 13.

2. Edmund Funai and Errol Norwitz, "Management of Normal Labor and Delivery," in *UpToDate*, ed. Ted W. Post (Waltham, MA: UpToDate, 2018).

3. Alexander M. Friedman, Cande V. Ananth, Eri Prendergast, Mary E. D'Alton, and Jason D. Wright, "Evaluation of Third-Degree and Fourth-Degree Laceration Rates as Quality Indicators," *Journal of Obstetric Gynecology* 125, no. 4 (April 2015): 927–37, https://www.ncbi.nlm.nih.gov/pubmed/25751203.

4. Michael Belfort, "Overview of Postpartum Hemorrhage," in *UpToDate*, ed. Ted W. Post (Waltham, MA: UpToDate, 2018).

5. Robert Resnik, "Clinical Features and Diagnosis of Placenta Accreta Spectrum," in *UpToDate*, ed. Ted W. Post (Waltham, MA: UpToDate, 2018).

6. Elizabeth R. Moore, Gene C. Anderson, Nils Bergman, and Therese Dowswell, "Early Skin-to-Skin Contact for Mothers and Their Healthy Newborn Infants," *Cochrane Database of Systematic Reviews*, issue 5, no. CD003519 (2012).

7. Pearl Houghteling and W. Allan Walker, "Why Is Initial Bacterial Colonization of the Intestine Important to the Infant's and Child's Health?" *Journal of Pediatric Gastroenterology and Nutrition* 60, no. 3 (2015): 294–307.

8. American College of Obstetricians and Gynecologists (ACOG), "Delayed Umbilical Cord Clamping after Birth," *Committee Opinion*, no. 684 (January 2017), https://www.acog.org/Clinical-Guidance-and-Publications/Committee-Opinions/Committee-on-Obstetric-Practice/Delayed-Umbilical-Cord-Clamping-After-Birth.

CHAPTER 9

1. Lauren Jansen, Martha Gibson, Betty Carlson Bowles, and Jane Leach, "First Do No Harm: Interventions during Childbirth," *Journal of Perinatal Education* 22, no. 2 (2013): 83–92.

2. Celeste Durnwald, "Diabetes Mellitus in Pregnancy: Screening and Diagnosis," in *UpToDate*, ed. Ted W. Post (Waltham, MA: UpToDate, 2018).

3. "Group B Strep Infection: GBS," American Pregnancy Association, last modified March 2, 2017, http://americanpregnancy.org/pregnancy-complications/group-b-strep-infection/.

4. "Group Beta Strep (GBS): Fast Facts," Centers for Disease Control and Prevention, accessed May 29, 2018, https://www.cdc.gov/groupbstrep/about/fast-facts.html.

5. Carol Baker, "Neonatal Group B Streptococcal Disease: Prevention," in *UpToDate*, ed. Ted W. Post (Waltham, MA: UpToDate, 2018).

6. Jennifer C. Stearns, Julia Simioni, Elizabeth Gunn, Helen McDonald, Alison C. Holloway, Lehana Thabane, Andrea Mousseau, Jonathan D. Schertzer, Elyanne M. Ratcliffe, Laura Rossi, Michael G. Surette, Katherine M. Morrison, and Eileen K. Hutton, "Intrapartum Antibiotics for GBS Prophylaxis Alter Colonization Patterns in the Early Infant Gut Microbiome of Low Risk Infants," *Scientific Reports* 7, no. 16527 (November 28, 2017).

7. Santiago Scasso, Joel Laufer, Grisel Rodriguez, Justo G. Alonso, and Claudio G. Sosa, "Vaginal Group B Streptococcus Status during Intrapartum Antibiotic Prophylaxis," *International Journal of Gynecology and Obstetrics* 129, no. 1 (April 2015): 9–12.

8. Rebecca Dekker, "The Evidence On: Group B Strep," Evidence Based Birth, last updated July 17, 2017, https://evidencebasedbirth.com/groupbstrep/.

9. Dekker, "Group B Strep."

10. "Obesity and Pregnancy," American College of Obstetricians and Gynecologists, last modified April 2016, https://www.acog.org/Patients/FAQs/Obesity-and-Pregnancy?IsMobileSet=false.

11. Declan Devane, Joan G. Lalor, Sean Daley, William McGuire, Anna Cuthbert, and Valerie Smith, "Cardiotocography versus Intermittent Auscultation of Fetal Heart on Admission of Labour Ward for Assessment of Fetal Wellbeing," *Cochrane Database of Systematic Reviews*, issue 1 (2012): 1–46.

12. M. Osterman and J. Martin, "Epidural and Spinal Anesthesia Use during Labor: 27-State Reporting Area, 2008," *National Vital Statistics Reports* 59, no. 5 (April 6, 2011), https://www.cdc.gov/nchs/data/nvsr/nvsr59/nvsr59_05.pdf.

13. Gilbert Grant, "Adverse Effects of Neuraxial Analgesia and Anesthesia for Obstetrics," in *UpToDate*, ed. Ted W. Post (Waltham, MA: UpToDate, 2018); C. L. Gurudatt, "Unintentional Dural Puncture and Postdural Puncture Headache—Can This Headache of the Patient as Well as the Anaesthesiologist Be Prevented?" *Indian Journal of Anesthesia* 58, no. 4 (2014): 385–87.

14. Gilbert Grant, "Adverse Effects of Neuraxial Analgesia and Anesthesia for Obstetrics," in *UpToDate*, ed. Ted W. Post (Waltham, MA: UpToDate, 2018).

15. Grant, "Adverse Effects."

16. Judith Rooks, "Safety and Risks of Nitrous Oxide Labor Analgesia: A Review," *Journal of Midwifery & Women's Health* 56, no. 6 (November/December 2011): 557–65.

17. Michael G. Richardson, Brandon M. Lopez, Curtis L. Baysinger, Matthew S. Shotwell, and David H. Chestnut, "Nitrous Oxide during Labor: Maternal Satisfaction Does Not Depend Exclusively on Analgesic Effectiveness," *Anesthesia & Analgesia* 124, no. 2 (February 2017): 548–53.

18. Roz Ullman, Lesley A. Smith, Ethel Burns, Rintaro Mori, and Therese Dowswell, "Parenteral Opioids for Maternal Pain Management in Labour," *Cochrane Database of Systematic Reviews*, issue 9, no. CD007396 (2010), https://doi.org/10.1002/14651858.CD007396.pub2.

19. M. Wegner and I. Bernstein, "Operative Vaginal Delivery," in *UpToDate*, ed. Ted W. Post (Waltham, MA: UpToDate, 2018).

20. Wegner and Bernstein, "Operative Vaginal Delivery."

21. Wegner and Bernstein, "Operative Vaginal Delivery."

22. L. Berkowitz and M. Foust-Wright, "Approach to Episiotomy," in *UpToDate*, ed. Ted W. Post (Waltham, MA: UpToDate, 2018).

23. Alexander M. Friedman, Cande V. Ananth, Eri Prendergast, Mary E. D'Alton, and Jason D. Wright, "Variation in and Factors Associated with Use of Episiotomy," *Journal of the American Medical Association* 313, no. 2 (2015): 197–99, https://doi.org/10.1001/jama.2014.14774.

24. Berkowitz and Foust-Wright, "Approach to Episiotomy."

25. Vincenzo Berghella, "Management of the Third Stage of Labor: Drug Therapy to Minimize Hemorrhage," in *UpToDate*, ed. Ted W. Post (Waltham, MA: UpToDate, 2018).

CHAPTER 10

1. Megan Davidson, "Experts in Birth: How Doulas Improve Outcomes for Birthing Women and Their Babies," in *Doulas and Intimate Labour: Boundaries, Bodies and Birth*, ed. Angela N. Castaneda and Julie Johnson Searcy (Bradford, ON: Demeter, 2015), 15–31.

CHAPTER 11

1. Michelle Osterman and Joyce A. Martin, "Recent Declines in Induction of Labor by Gestational Age," *NCHS Data Brief*, no. 155 (June 2014), https://www.cdc.gov/nchs/products/databriefs/db155.htm.

2. T. A. Bruckner, Y. W. Cheng, and A. B. Caughey, "Increased Neonatal Mortality among Normal-Weight Births beyond 41 Weeks of Gestation in California," *American Journal of Obstetrics & Gynecology* 199, no. 4 (2008); Michael Y. Divon, Bengt Haglund, Henry Nisell, Petra Olausson Otterblad, and Magnus Westgren, "Fetal and Neonatal Mortality in the Poster Pregnancy: The Impact of Gestational Age and Fetal Growth Restriction," *American Journal of Obstetrics & Gynecology* 178, no. 4 (1998); G. B. Feldman, "Prospective Risk of Stillbirth," *Obstetrics & Gynecology* 79, no. 4 (1992).

3. Erika R. Cheng, Eugene R. Declercq, Candice Belanoff, Naomi E. Stotland, and Ronald E. Iverson, "Labor and Delivery Experiences of Mothers with Suspected Large Babies," *Maternal and Child Health Journal* 19, no. 12 (December 2016): 2578–86; Julia Milner and Jane Arezina, "The Accuracy of Ultrasound Estimation of Fetal Weight in Comparison to Birth Weight: A Systematic Review," *Ultrasound* 26, no. 1 (February 2018); Roni Caryn Rabin, "When a Big Baby Isn't So Big," *New York Times*, January 11, 2016, https://well.blogs.nytimes.com/2016/01/11/high-birth-weight-predictions-are-often-inaccurate/.

4. N. Borders, R. Lawton, and S. R. Martin, "A Clinical Audit of the Number of Vaginal Examinations in Labor: A NOVEL Idea," *Journal of Midwifery & Women's Health* 57, no. 2 (March/April 2012): 139–44; William Scorza, "Management of Prelabor Rupture of the Fetal Membranes at Term," in *UpToDate*, ed. Ted W. Post (Waltham, MA: UpToDate, 2018); World Health Organization (Technical Working Group), "Care in Normal Birth: A Practical Guide," *Birth* 24, no. 2 (June 1997): 121–23.

5. Scorza, "Management of Prelabor Rupture."

6. William Grobman, "Techniques for Ripening the Unfavorable Cervix prior to Induction," in *UpToDate*, ed. Ted W. Post (Waltham, MA: UpToDate, 2018).

7. Grobman, "Techniques."

8. William Grobman, "Induction of Labor with Oxytocin," in *UpToDate*, ed. Ted W. Post (Waltham, MA: UpToDate, 2018).

9. Grobman, "Induction of Labor"; George A. Macones, Alison Cahill, David M. Stamilio, and Anthony O. Odibo, "The Efficacy of Early Amniotomy in Nulliparous Labor Induction: A Randomized Controlled Trial," *American Journal of Obstetrics & Gynecology* 207, no. 5 (November 2012): 403.

10. M. Boulvain, C. Stan, and O. Irion, "Membrane Sweeping for Induction of Labour," *Cochrane Database of Systematic Reviews*, issue 1, no. CD000451 (2005), https://doi.org/10.1002/14651858.CD000451.pub2.

11. O. Al-Kuran, L. Al-Mehaisen, H. Bawadi, S. Beitawi, and Z. Amarin, "The Effect of Late Pregnancy Consumption of Date Fruit on Labour and Delivery," *Journal of Obstetrics and Gynaecology* 31, no. 1 (2011): 29–31; Masoumeh Kordi, Fatemeh Aghaei Meybodi, Fatemeh Tara, Mohsen Nemati, and Mohammad Taghi Shakeri, "The Effect of Late Pregnancy Consumption of Date Fruit on Cervical Ripening in Nulliparous Women," *Journal of Midwifery and Reproductive Health* 2, no. 3 (July 2014): 150–56; Nuguelis Razali, Siti Hayati Mohd Nahwari, Sofiah Sulaiman, and Jamiyah Hassan, "Date Fruit Consumption at Term: Effect on Length of Gestation, Labour and Delivery," *Journal of Obstetrics and Gynaecology* 37, no. 5 (July 2017): 595–600.

12. P. Middleton, E. Shepherd, and C. A. Crowther, "Induction of Labour for Improving Birth Outcomes for Women at or beyond Term," *Cochrane Database of Systematic Reviews*, issue 5, no. CD004945 (May 2018), https://doi.org/10.1002/14651858.CD004945.pub4; Ekaterina Mishanina, Ewelina Rogozinska, Tej Thatthi, Rehan Uddin-Khan, Khalid S. Khan, and Catherine Meads, "Use of Labour Induction and

Risk of Cesarean Delivery: A Systematic Review and Meta-analysis," *Canadian Medical Association Journal* 186, no. 9 (June 2014): 665–73.

CHAPTER 12

1. Torri Metz, "Choosing the Route of Delivery after Cesarean Birth," in *UpTo-Date*, ed. Ted W. Post (Waltham, MA: UpToDate, 2018).

2. Metz, "Choosing the Route of Delivery."

3. Mark Landon and Heather Frey, "Uterine Rupture: After Previous Cesarean Delivery," in *UpToDate*, ed. Ted W. Post (Waltham, MA: UpToDate, 2018).

4. Metz, "Choosing the Route of Delivery"; Landon and Frey, "Uterine Rupture."

5. Metz, "Choosing the Route of Delivery."

6. Metz, "Choosing the Route of Delivery."

7. American College of Obstetricians and Gynecologist (ACOG), "Placenta Accreta," *Committee Opinion*, no. 529 (July 2012, reaffirmed 2017); Katheryne Downes, Stefanie N. Hinkle, Lindsey A. Sjaarda, Paul S. Albert, and Katherine L. Grantz, "Prior Prelabor or Intrapartum Cesarean Delivery and Risk of Placenta Previa," *American Journal of Obstetrics and Gynecology* 212, no. 5 (May 2015): 669; Robert Resnik and Robert Silver, "Clinical Features and Diagnosis of Placenta Accreta Spectrum (Placenta Accreta, Increta, and Percreta)," in *UpToDate*, ed. Ted W. Post (Waltham, MA: UpToDate, 2018).

8. Vincenzo Berghella, "Caesarean Delivery: Postoperative Issues," in *UpToDate*, ed. Ted W. Post (Waltham, MA: UpToDate, 2018); Metz, "Choosing the Route of Delivery."

9. Mark B. Landon, Sharon Leindecker, Catherine Y. Spong, John C. Hauth, Steven Bloom, Michael W. Varner, Atef H. Moawad, Steve N. Caritis, Margaret Harper, Ronald J. Wapner, Yoram Sorokin, Menachem Miodovnik, Marshall Carpenter, Alan M. Peaceman, Mary Jo O'Sullivan, Baha M. Sibai, Oded Langer, John M. Thorp, Susan M. Ramin, Brian M. Mercer, and Steven G. Gabbe, "The MFMU Cesarean Registry: Factors Affecting the Success of Trial of Labor after Previous Cesarean Delivery," *American Journal of Obstetrics and Gynecology* 193, no. 3 (September 2005): 1016–23; Metz, "Choosing the Route of Delivery."

10. Metz, "Choosing the Route of Delivery."

11. American College of Obstetricians and Gynecologists (ACOG) and the Society for Maternal-Fetal Medicine (SMFM), "Safe Prevention of the Primary Cesarean Delivery," *Obstetric Care Consensus*, no. 1 (March 2014, reaffirmed 2016): 13.

12. Erika R. Cheng, , Eugene R. Declercq, Candice Belanoff, Naomi E. Stotland, and Ronald E. Iverson, "Labor and Delivery Experiences of Mothers with Suspected Large Babies," *Maternal and Child Health Journal* 19, no. 12 (December 2016): 2578–86; Julia Milner and Jane Arezina, "The Accuracy of Ultrasound Estimation of

Fetal Weight in Comparison to Birth Weight: A Systematic Review," *Ultrasound* 26, no. 1 (February 2018).

13. American College of Obstetricians and Gynecologists (ACOG), "Planned Home Birth," *Committee Opinion*, no. 697 (April 2017, reaffirmed 2018), https://www.acog. org/Clinical-Guidance-and-Publications/Committee-Opinions/Committee-on-Obstet- ric-Practice/Planned-Home-Birth.

14. Torri Metz, "Trial of Labor after Cesarean Delivery: Intrapartum Management," in *UpToDate*, ed. Ted W. Post (Waltham, MA: UpToDate, 2018).

CHAPTER 13

1. Joyce A. Martin, Brady E. Hamilton, Michelle J. K. Osterman, Anne K. Driscoll, and Patrick Drake, "Births: Final Data for 2016," *National Vital Statistics Reports* 67, no. 1 (January 31, 2018): 9, https://www.cdc.gov/nchs/data/nvsr/nvsr67/nvsr67_01. pdf.

2. Stephen Chasen, "Twins Pregnancy: Prenatal Issues," in *UpToDate*, ed. Ted W. Post (Waltham, MA: UpToDate, 2018).

3. Chasen, "Twins Pregnancy: Prenatal Issues."

4. Chasen, "Twins Pregnancy: Prenatal Issues."

5. Chasen, "Twins Pregnancy: Prenatal Issues."

6. C. A. Crowther, "Hospitalisation and Bed Rest for Multiple Pregnancy," *Cochrane Database of Systematic Reviews*, issue 7, no. CD000110 (2010); Katharina da Silva Lopes, Yo Takemoto, Erika Ota, Shinji Tanigaki, and Rintaro Mori, "Bed Rest with and without Hospitalisation in Multiple Pregnancy for Improving Perinatal Outcomes," *Cochrane Database of Systematic Reviews*, issue 3, no. CD012031 (2017); A. C. Sciscione, "Maternal Activity Restriction and the Prevention of Preterm Birth," *American Journal of Obstetrics and Gynecology* 202, no. 3 (2010): 232.e1; Chasen, "Twins Pregnancy: Prenatal Issues.".

7. Stephen Chasen and Frank Chervenak, "Twin Pregnancy: Labor and Delivery," in *UpToDate*, ed. Ted W. Post (Waltham, MA: UpToDate, 2018).

8. American College of Obstetricians and Gynecologists (ACOG) and the Society for Maternal-Fetal Medicine (SMFM), "Safe Prevention of the Primary Cesarean Delivery," *Obstetric Care Consensus*, no. 1 (March 2014, reaffirmed 2016): 13; Chasen and Chervenak, "Twin Pregnancy: Labor and Delivery."

CHAPTER 14

1. "Births—Method of Delivery," National Center for Health Statistics, CDC, last modified March 31, 2017, https://www.cdc.gov/nchs/fastats/delivery.htm.

2. Eugene Declercq, Fay Menacker, and Marian MacDorman, "Maternal Risk Profiles and the Primary Cesarean Rate in the United States, 1991–2002," *American Journal of Obstetrics and Gynecology* 95, no. 5 (May 2006): 867–72; American College of Obstetricians and Gynecologists (ACOG) and the Society for Maternal-Fetal Medicine (SMFM), "Safe Prevention of the Primary Cesarean Delivery," *Obstetric Care Consensus*, no. 1 (March 2014, reaffirmed 2016): 3.

3. American College of Obstetricians and Gynecologists (ACOG), "Cesarean Delivery on Maternal Request," *Committee Opinion*, no. 559 (April 2013, reaffirmed 2017).

4. Charles Lockwood and Karen Russo-Stieglitz, "Placenta Previa: Epidemiology, Clinical Features, Diagnosis, Morbidity and Mortality," in *UpToDate*, ed. Ted W. Post (Waltham, MA: UpToDate, 2018).

5. Charles Lockwood and Karen Russo-Stieglitz, "Velamentous Umbilical Cord Insertion and Vasa Previa," in *UpToDate*, ed. Ted W. Post (Waltham, MA: UpToDate, 2018).

6. Lockwood and Russo-Stieglitz, "Velamentous Umbilical Cord Insertion."

7. G. Justus Hofmeyr, "Overview of Issues Related to Breech Presentation," in *UpToDate*, ed. Ted W. Post (Waltham, MA: UpToDate, 2018).

8. Stephen Chasen and Frank Chervenak, "Twin Pregnancy: Labor and Delivery," in *UpToDate*, ed. Ted W. Post (Waltham, MA: UpToDate, 2018).

9. Shayna N. Conner, Juliana C. Verticchio, Methodius G. Tuuli, Anthony O. Odibo, George A. Macones, and Alison G. Cahill, "Maternal Obesity and Risk of Post-Cesarean Wound Complications," *American Journal of Perinatology* 31, no. 4 (2014): 299–304; Richard Porreco, "Cesarean Delivery of the Obese Woman," in *UpToDate*, ed. Ted W. Post (Waltham, MA: UpToDate, 2018).

10. Cande Ananth and Wendy L. Kinzler, "Placental Abruption: Pathophysiology, Clinical Features, Diagnosis, and Consequences," in *UpToDate*, ed. Ted W. Post (Waltham, MA: UpToDate, 2018).

11. Melissa Bush, Keith Eddleman, and Victoria Belogolovkin, "Umbilical Cord Prolapse," in *UpToDate*, ed. Ted W. Post (Waltham, MA: UpToDate, 2018).

12. George Molina, Thomas G. Weiser, Stuart R. Lipsitz, Micaela M. Esquivel, Tarsicio Uribe-Leitz, Tej Azad, Neel Shah, Katherine Semrau, William R. Berry, Atul A. Gawande, and Alex B. Haynes, "Relationship between Cesarean Delivery Rate and Maternal and Neonatal Mortality," *Journal of the American Medical Association* 314, no. 21 (2015): 2263–70; World Health Organization, "Appropriate Technology for Birth," *Lancet* 2, no. 8452 (1985): 436–37.

13. ACOG and SMFM, "Safe Prevention of the Primary Cesarean Delivery."

14. ACOG and SMFM, "Safe Prevention of the Primary Cesarean Delivery."

15. Erika R. Cheng, Eugene R. Declercq, Candice Belanoff, Naomi E. Stotland, and Ronald E. Iverson, "Labor and Delivery Experiences of Mothers with Suspected Large Babies," *Maternal and Child Health Journal* 19, no. 12 (December 2016): 2578–86; Julia Milner and Jane Arezina, "The Accuracy of Ultrasound Estimation of Fetal Weight

in Comparison to Birth Weight: A Systematic Review," *Ultrasound* 26, no. 1 (February 2018); Roni Caryn Rabin, "When a Big Baby Isn't So Big," *New York Times*, January 11, 2016, https://well.blogs.nytimes.com/2016/01/11/high-birth-weight-predictions-are-often-inaccurate/.

16. Meaghan A. Leddy, Michael L. Power, and Jay Schulkin, "The Impact of Maternal 'Obesity' on Maternal and Fetal Health." *Reviews in Obstetrics & Gynecology* 1, no. 4 (2008):175.

17. ACOG and SMFM, "Safe Prevention of the Primary Cesarean Delivery."

18. G. Justus Hofmeyr, "External Cephalic Version," in *UpToDate*, ed. Ted W. Post (Waltham, MA: UpToDate, 2018).

19. G. Justus Hofmeyr, "Delivery of the Fetus in Breech Presentation," in *UpToDate*, ed. Ted W. Post (Waltham, MA: UpToDate, 2018).

20. Hofmeyr, "Fetus in Breech Presentation."

21. Irene Yang, "The Infant Microbiome: Implications for Infant Health and Neurocognitive Development," *Nursing Research* 65, no. 1 (2016): 76–88; Jane Brody, "Exposing Infants to Micro-organisms," *New York Times*, February 6, 2018, D5.

ACKNOWLEDGMENTS

I imagined this book for many years before I ever considered writing it. My friend Lisa Jean Moore gave me the shove I needed to begin writing and without her, I'm not sure I would have ever taken my desire for this book and turned it into something. She was my writing buddy and biggest cheerleader, mentoring and guiding me through every step of this project. My gratitude is never ending.

C. Ray Borck was not so sure about having a doula in his writing group or reading an entire book about birth, but he always returned the best edits and feedback, filled with exclamation marks, emojis, and love. His lack of knowledge about anything birth turned out to be priceless. Thank you for being a friend.

My agent Anjali Singh (Ayesha Pande Literary) was truly my book doula. She believed in me and kept me positive, answered all my questions, put up with all my protests, and advocated for me and for this project. Your support has been invaluable and so appreciated.

My clients and friends have given so generously to make this book possible—granting me permission to share parts of their stories, answering all my questions about what made their births positive experiences, sharing their photographs, and enthusiastically supporting me the whole way. I give so much thanks for families trusting me with their intimate moments and for always feeling like I lucked out and ended up with the absolute best job in the whole world.

Andrea, Jill, Mary, and Jess, as well as my wonderful editor Suzanne Staszak-Silva, all offered valuable feedback and edits on drafts of this book; their assistance was so appreciated. Stephanie and Sarah cheered me on, talked through my ideas, and insisted throughout that writing this book was a good idea, even when I had moments of being less convinced.

My family has put up with the long, slow process of me writing this book between the prenatal and postpartum visits, births, and client calls that already fill so much of my days. I'm thankful for their good spirits and generosity over these last years as I missed out on games and adventures in order to finish another chapter.

Shawn has always believed in me and supported me, encouraged me, and been proud of me. The impact of this in my life, and on this project, is immeasurable. In this project he was especially heroic, reading every word I wrote and patiently correcting all my commas.

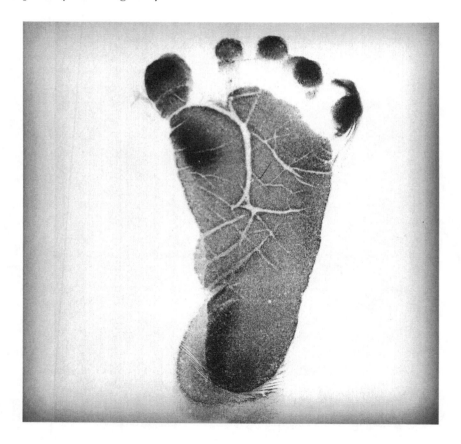

INDEX

pulse rate: monitoring, 139, 142; of
newborn, 130
pushing: with epidural, 125; during
labor, 125–27; positions for, 126;
support during, 125

racism, during pregnancy, xxiv
rape crisis advocate, x
Raphael, Dana, 91, 101
rectal pressure, during labor, 123
red blood cell, protein in, 139
reflex response, of newborn, 130
respiratory effort, of newborn, 130
resting posture, 131
resuscitation gear, 34
retained placenta, 128
Rh factor, 139
Rhogam, 139, 183
"ring of fire," 126
risk: of birth center, 23–25; bleeding, 59,
98, 127, 142, 271; blood clotting,
59, 139, 220, 242, 257; of Cesarean
birth, 242; during childbirth, xxii;
of circumcision, 259–60; doula and,
103; of induction, 201; medication,
59; for MFM doctor, 58–60;
midwives and, 78–80, 84; with
multiple birth, 218–20; obstetric,
32; of placenta attachment, 206;
pregnancy, 57–58, 78–80, 103;
during pregnancy, xxiii, 57; with
twins, 218–20; of VBAC, 204–8
rubella, 139

safety, of homebirth, 32
saline lock, 144
scar: thickness of, 205; tissue, 206
scopolamine, 11
"seed," 244
seizure disorder, 59, 78
sepsis, 143

sex: bed rest and, 219; bleeding and,
121; after childbirth, 271; hepatitis B
and, 258; for inducing labor, 4, 196;
infection and, 142–43, 257; mucus
plug and, 114; of twins, 218
sex chromosomes, 139
sexual abuse, 235
shaking, during labor, 121–23
siblings: birth plan for, 39–40; at
homebirth, 30, 30–31, 34, 39–40
sickness, morning, 219
silver nitrate, 12
sitz bath, 270
skin color, of newborn, 130
skin to skin contact, 129, 143; after
Cesarean birth, 234, 243; low blood
sugar and, 259
sleep, twilight, 253
SMFM. See The Society for Maternal-
Fetal Medicine
social worker, in NICU, 262
The Society for Maternal-Fetal Medicine
(SMFM), 95, 239; Cesarean birth
and, 240
sodium chloride, 144
sodium lactate, 144
sonographer, 3, 218
spinal headache, 154
spiritual adviser, on birth team, 49
Stadol, 157
station, 109
sterile drape, 243
sterile water injections (SWI), 159–60
stethoscope, 146
stool softener, 269
stretch marks, 272
"struggle less," 131
sufentanil, 151
"sunny-side up," 109
support group: in-person, 263; online,
65, 263; postpartum, 272

ABOUT THE AUTHOR

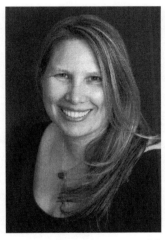

Megan Davidson, PhD, is a doula and child-birth educator practicing in New York City with over ten years' experience supporting pregnant people and new families with every type of birth plan and preference. She believes in helping people have respectful, informed, positive experiences of childbirth and has attended nearly six hundred births and worked with more than twelve hundred families post-partum. Megan has published ethnographic research on how doulas improve outcomes for pregnant people and their babies, as well as essays on both fat phobia in prenatal care and transgender activism, and she is regularly quoted as an expert on a wide range of childbirth and postpartum topics in national media, including the *LA Times*, *The Today Show*, and Fox News' *Headline Health*, among others. Megan and her family live in Clinton Hill, Brooklyn.